The American Society of Internal Medicine gratefully acknowledges the support of the following organizations for their contributions toward the publication of this book:

CIBA-GEIGY Corporation, Pharmaceuticals Division
Hoechst-Roussel Pharmaceuticals Inc.
Mead Johnson Pharmaceutical Division
Merck Sharp & Dohme
Pfizer Pharmaceuticals
William H. Rorer, Inc.
Ross Laboratories Division of Abbott Laboratories

The Story of
The American Society of
Internal Medicine
1956-1981

ASPIRATION & ACHIEVEMENT

William Campbell Felch, M.D. and
Clyde C. Greene, Jr., M.D.

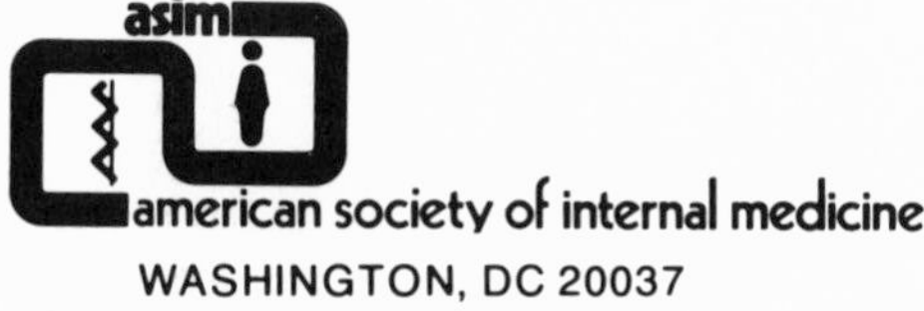

WASHINGTON, DC 20037

Published and distributed by the
American Society of Internal Medicine
2550 M St., NW, Suite 620
Washington, DC 20037

Library of Congress Cataloging in Publication Data

Felch, William et al.

Aspiration & Achievement

8109 810814

LCCN 81-69266

ISBN 0-9607006-0-9 Case Bound
ISBN 0-9607006-1-7 Perfect Bound

Printed in the United States of America
Cover Design: Eileen Divine

Table of Contents

President's Comments

It is altogether fitting that a major professional specialty organization should take cognizance of its 25th birthday by commissioning the writing of a history of that interesting, and sometimes turbulent, quarter of a century.

In 1980, ASIM's Board of Trustees, aware that the silver jubilee was only a year away, took action to approve the creation of such a chronicle. And to write it the Board asked two old ASIM hands, who between them had been in positions of influence in the Society through the entire span of years from 1956 to 1981.

Clyde C. Greene, Jr., MD, attended the Founders Meeting in April 1956, became the fledgling ASIM's assistant secretary-treasurer two years later, and its secretary-treasurer—through some financially strained early years—in 1959, a position he held for nine years. In 1968 he was selected president-elect and the following year became the Society's 13th president. Completing his past presidency in 1971, he was appointed editor of *The Internist* and continued in that capacity until 1975. The list of Clyde's contributions to ASIM during those 19 years of stewardship is remarkable, not only in major policy innovations, but also, especially, in countless meticulous bits of attention to day-to-day operational detail.

William Campbell Felch, MD, first attended an ASIM meeting, almost by chance, in 1962. A year later, he was a member of the Medical Services Committee, and a year after that, he was chairman of the Health Insurance Committee. In 1968 he became a Trustee and in 1972 was elected president-elect, becoming ASIM's 17th president in 1973. He, in turn, after completing his year as past president, became editor of *The Internist,* a position he still holds. His various contributions to ASIM over the last 18 years have been—to use one of his favorite expressions—both broad and deep. They have included consideration of the conceptual—see his series of presidential columns on "The Role of the Internist"—and involvement with the practical—as chairman of a host of ASIM councils, committees and task forces.

These two men have devoted countless hours to the creation of this history of ASIM's first 25 years. It is my belief that it serves as a significant contribution to the understanding of this remarkable organization.

John F. Farrington, MD
President, 1980-81

President-Elect's Comments

If history is but the prologue to the future, and if the future seems to resemble if not repeat the past, then there is much to be learned from a retelling of ASIM's first quarter century. Perhaps the most important revelation will come from the display of the Society's source of strength. You will come to see, as you read of ASIM's past deeds, that they were fashioned by thoughtful, gentle men and women who shared an inner, steel-like quality in their sense of purpose: to be the advocate for practicing internists and their patients.

Every successful organization can be placed at some point along the spectrum of Vitality. First, there is the Survival phase when all resources are devoted to establishing simple existence. This is followed by a Profit phase when some of the returns can be put aside to establish the future security of the organization. The next step is generally a Growth phase, in which the organization seeks to expand to reach its maximum potential. Finally, in the case of truly successful organizations, there emerges an involvement in the Greater Society, a phase in which energies can be devoted to projects and concerns reflecting the clear needs of society as a whole; such projects no longer relate solely to the survival, profit or growth of the organization.

ASIM is now well past concerns about survival and profit, and, in my opinion, is deeply involved in its own growth and stretching toward the needs of the greater society. The next quarter century will bring its own judgment about those efforts, but we are rich in opportunities with no reason to fear that our primary resource—practicing internists—will run dry.

There is much to learn from our past. As the historian, Thucydides, said over two thousand years ago, ". . . the bravest are surely those who have the clearest vision of what is before them, glory and danger alike, and yet notwithstanding go out to meet it." Let all internists gather under the ASIM banner to meet the challenge, for it is clearly our heritage and it may well be our destiny.

Lonnie R. Bristow, MD
President-Elect, 1980-81

Authors' Note

To some extent, this is a conventional history, in that it records the events that took place during ASIM's first 25 years and the people who made them happen. But readers looking for a precise chronology of everything that took place since 1956 or for mention of every person involved, will have to look elsewhere, perhaps in the archives at the Society's headquarters office.

Our aim has been to write something different than a dry record of people and events, something that is closer to a memoir—or perhaps a personality profile—of this unusual Society. Our approach has been to think of ASIM as though it were a human being, and we have tried to portray how it was born, the environment in which it spent its infancy, its first struggles to achieve an identity, its sometimes turbulent growth and development, and its gradual evolution into the mature organization of today.

To help us in adding substance to this conceptual strategy, we called on the people who created the ASIM persona. We prepared a master list of leaders, past and present, national and local, and asked them—through a questionnaire—to recount their memories of what they caused to happen and what happened to them that was inspiring, troubling—or amusing.

It must be admitted that it took a second mailing to get some laggards to respond. And a few others saw fit to dispense with the survey form in order to submit a narrative account of their version of history. But the final returns were impressive—testimony perhaps to the compulsiveness of good internists, but more likely a tribute to the devotion that involvement in Society activities breeds: no less than 84, or 67%, sent in some kind of report.

A mound of material—factual, sentimental, anecdotal, opinionated—was thus generated. In addition, there were past minutes of Board meetings, past issues of *The Internist,* and past reports of task forces/councils/advisory groups/committees. The difficult winnowing process was conducted with the principal criterion being to eliminate anything that did not add to the establishment of the ASIM persona.

The process of writing came next. One of us (WCF) prepared first drafts of chapters. These were then "cleaned up" (by the estimable Connie Schantz, staff managing editor, without whose hours of devoted work this account would never have been accomplished) and then edited again by the other one of us (CCG, Jr.).

We hope that the end product, *Aspiration & Achievement,* will afford some pleasure to readers, both to the many individuals who contributed in one way or another to the growth of the ASIM child, and the even greater number of rank-and-file members who may find in these pages an understanding of what has made their organization the remarkable Society it is.

William Campbell Felch, MD
Clyde C. Greene, Jr., MD

VOLUME I

The Early Years

Accouchement and Activation

Aphorism: Grand Rounds

They might have been conducting grand rounds or participating in a clinico-pathologic conference, these forty-five internists gathered in Los Angeles from twenty-one states, two Canadian Provinces, the District of Columbia and the territory of Hawaii (which, in April 1956, was still three years from statehood).

The Californians present, acting in their capacity both as hosts for the occasion and as members of the largest and oldest state society of internal medicine, made the formal case presentation. First came the history: the public has failed to understand what internal medicine is and what internists do. Then came the physical examination: health insurance payment schedules largely overlook the services characteristic of internal medicine.

Next came the differential diagnosis: The manifestations of the affliction vary somewhat in different parts of the country. Finally, the 45 attendees agreed on a consensus diagnosis: the lack of recognition of the worth of internists is a problem of national dimensions.

It did not take long for the founding group to decide on proper therapy: a national organization is needed to serve the interests of internists and their patients.

A motion was made and passed unanimously in support of the proposed therapy. Preliminary strategies were agreed on for developing and implementing a treatment plan.

Thus was born the American Society of Internal Medicine.

1

The General Environment

American Ambience

The events that took place on that noteworthy day in 1956 are clear enough. The words that were said have been transcribed and the outcome—the unanimous vote to form an American Society of Internal Medicine—has been preserved for us. Reading between the dry lines of the transcript, one can sense some collective feelings: certainly, a pervasive aura of purpose and mission; to some degree, an atmosphere of enthusiasm, even excitement; and, above all, a sense of mutual resolve to get on with the job ahead.

But events such as these do not take place suddenly, appearing out of a void. Nor do such collective feelings arise spontaneously, fired by some whimsical internal combustion. What circumstances led up to the meeting on April 15, 1956? What mood prevailed in the country? What was happening in the health arena? Where did internal medicine fit into the jigsaw puzzle of medical care? What problems needed solving that required the collective involvement of internists throughout the nation?

Looking back 25 years through the rose-colored lenses of memory, we tend to think of the fifties as a placid era, basically a happy one. The scars from depression years were fading; youngsters were growing up who had not lived through its degradations. The new affluent society was firmly in place. War seemed to be a thing of the past: the second World War had been over for more than a decade and the Korean conflict, for more than three years. There was room for optimism that the new United Nations might somehow preserve the peace.

The family unit was flourishing, even taking into account the sugar coating TV gave it. Individual citizens, at least most of them, faced the future with equanimity, even outright confidence. There were some signs—balm to collective guilty conscience—that the deprived members of our society would at last get a fair shake: the Supreme Court had ordered school desegregation in 1954 and the U.S. Congress was working on civil rights legislation that would become law in 1957.

The fifties was a decade exemplified by some of the personal qualities of its principal figure—Dwight D. Eisenhower. Perhaps there was no brilliance, but there certainly was steadfastness. If he failed to stimulate intellectual ferment, he did inspire trust. His personal warmth and homespun dignity gave the people sufficient reason to vote for him. In

1956, finishing off his first term as president, he took on and beat a redoubtable political personality, the wryly intellectual Adlai Stevenson.

There was one aspect of the Eisenhower era, however, that was anything but placid. Science and technology were booming, caught up in a riptide of change. The scope of scientific achievement was expanding dramatically—especially at the opposite ends of the physical spectrum. At the cellular pole, the atom had been split in the forties and two atom bombs had brought World War II to an end. At the celestial end, new technology, especially in rocket propulsion, was making feasible man's age-old dream of exploring space.

Despite some ambivalence and misgivings, most people worshipped at the shrine of science and technology. At the basic level, the hard sciences of physics and mathematics were thriving and their role model was Albert Einstein. At the applied level, it was electronics and engineering, bringing us the wonders of color television, fast cars, and data processing computers. The Nobel Prize in 1956 was awarded for the development of the transistor.

The softer sciences also joined the technologic bandwagon. Economists used econometric measures to project where our economy was heading (although one could always find two economists who, using the same data, would somehow arrive at opposite conclusions). Political science turned to demographers and pollsters to determine what a candidate's political stance should be—although precision of the data sometimes seemed to have less to do with winning or losing than did the candidate's personality as projected on the TV screen. Even hard-headed businessmen took a leaf from the scientist's notebook, bringing in efficiency experts to give them advice about how to deal with personnel, how to enhance productivity, and how to manage by objective.

The people's love affair with science and technology was especially visible in the field of the basic biologic sciences and their application—health care. There was growing optimism that the scientific method could pay immense dividends in terms of improving the public's health. The successful development by Jonas Salk of an effective polio vaccine in 1954 ended that scourge (universally feared by parents) and seemed to put nearly the last nail in the coffin of infectious diseases. If polio could be eradicated, surely science could soon cure the common cold and other such troublesome afflictions. And with acute illnesses eliminated, science should logically be equally capable of vanquishing the dread degenerative diseases such as heart disease, stroke and, above all, cancer.

Where once illness and death were simply part of the human condition, expected events for every family to accept with fatalism, now there was reasonable hope that medical science could prevent or even eliminate sickness and could postpone death until a ripe old age.

Public confidence in the efficacy of science was also manifested in government. Health had achieved Cabinet-level status in 1953 when President Eisenhower created the Department of Health, Education and Welfare and appointed a woman, Oveta Culp Hobby, to run it. The National Institutes of Health, existing in modest form since 1935, was now located on a gleaming new campus in Bethesda and was ready to crank up a partnership with the nation's medical schools to promote the advancement of medical research. Technology also showed up in other places on the health care scene. Helped by government funds under the Hill-Burton program, shining new hospitals were built all over the country, full of modern surgical suites, marvelous new radiological machines, and efficient new laboratory gadgets.

These manifestations of medical science and the day-to-day successes with which they were crowned were not hidden from the eyes of the public. President Eisenhower's heart attack in 1955 and his surgically treated attack of ileitis in 1956 were recounted in the mass media in specific (some people thought far too explicit), clinical detail. Magazines found that anything with medical content had a ready audience. Newspapers printed regular columns devoted to clinical and/or research subjects. Among TV's most popular personalities were two physicians named Kildare and Casey.

Inevitably, the demand for medical care increased. People went to the doctor in droves and many communities had too few doctors on hand to deal comfortably with the surging demand. Those beleaguered doctors, bone-weary and harassed, were beginning to look for help—in the form of physician extenders and more efficient methods of office management—in handling their patient loads.

Medical care, once a low priority item on the national agenda, one which our hardy pioneer ancestors had disdained or learned to do without, was becoming a major thread in the fabric of everyday life. Medical care, the politicians figured out, was no longer a luxury or a privilege; it ranked right up there with food, clothing, shelter and education as one of our citizens' natural and inalienable rights. Medical care, the orators agreed, of optimal quality and at a reasonable price, should be accessible to all Americans.

2

The Professional Environment
Arenas and Allegiances

Doctors returning to practice from World War II (or from its Korean aftershock in the early fifties), as well as those just starting out in practice, found themselves in a radically evolving environment, one in which the delivery of medical care kept changing dramatically.

The scientific explosion and increasing public expectations about the benefits of health care produced a corresponding increase in the demand for medical care services. One result was growing pressures on physicians to deliver more services. Doctors inevitably got busier than they had been before, at times busier than they wanted to be.

Rising expectations also meant that people would look for the best care possible. The trend seemed inexorable: people would no longer settle for the jack-of-all-trades care offered by the general practitioner; it became fashionable to "go to a specialist." What was later to be labeled "primary care"—that amalgam of first contact, continuing, personal care—turned from the exclusive domain of the general practitioner and became an extra stock in trade for pediatricians, obstetrician-gynecologists and, especially, internists.

Expectations for better care also meant a willingness to pay higher prices for it. Although patients might willingly pay more for an occasional office visit to a specialist, an increasing part of the medical care dollar—especially for hospital care—was being paid through the insurance or prepayment mechanism. This meant that doctor-specialists had to convince not only their patients of the propriety of their fees; they would have to educate—or persuade—the third-party payors and their bureaucracies. Higher fees had to be justified—in terms of quality of care rendered or at least of the time spent with the patient—and this required a separate nomenclature system to distinguish, say, the office visit as delivered by an internist from that given by the GP or the surgeon.

All of these changes in the environment of physicians' practices had to be dealt with in some way. Individual doctors, finding it nearly impossible to resolve problems on their own, turned to collective organizations to negotiate for them. The traditional professional hierarchies—AMA, state medical associations, county medical societies—still carried the principal brunt of handling social, economic and political problems for doctors. But the rise of specialization was creating different loyalties, a new tendency for doctors to turn to their specialty organization to help with problems. The American College of Surgeons had worked hard to upgrade the identity and prestige of the well-trained surgeon (while less explicitly downgrading the surgical competence of GPs). Similarly, the American College of Obstetrics and Gynecology had gone to bat for its skilled member specialists, again implying the contrast with the less thoroughly trained GP.

The influences that were provoking change in the environment for the medical profession as a whole were producing especially marked effects on practitioners of internal medicine. Indeed, it can be said safely that the fifties were a time of "identity crisis" for internal medicine.

For one thing, the erosion of general practice had special implications to internists. On the one hand, the traditional relationship had consisted of the internist serving as a consultant to the GP, helping him with problem cases as a diagnostician. As the numbers of GPs diminished, so did the number of referrals to internist consultants.

On the other hand, the new role of the internist—to provide both first contact and continuing personal care to patients—was in direct competition with the generalist function of the GP. By the mid-fifties, most communities of any size had a number of internists offering their services to the public. Family practitioners (FPs) had not yet appeared on the scene and the dwindling numbers of GPs, still struggling to be all things to all people, were too busy with their remaining loyal patients to care much if some less loyal ones went down the street to the new internist in town. Indeed, in many communities, the two types of physicians lived in a kind of symbiosis, the internist having his own practice while at the same time serving as a consultant for the GP's more difficult cases.*

But not every citizen had the knowledge to make the switch to internal medicine promptly. The truth is that a sizable portion of the populace did not know what an internist was or what an internist did. To many, the name was confused with intern, that fledgling physician

*This is not the place to chronicle in detail the determined efforts by GP leaders to overcome the diminished numbers and status of their members. The change in name to family practice, the decision to identify it as a specialty, the creation of a board, the development of a three-year residency program, all were part of a concerted and well planned effort to put life back into a dying breed. The effort has met with considerable success. The new family physician has taken his place at the banquet table of medical care delivery. And the organizations representing him—the American Academy of Family Physicians for educational matters and the American Board of Family Practice for certifying and recertifying its diplomates—have taken their place in the hegemony of organized medicine and have exerted a strong voice in professional, social, economic, and political circles. Some critics have argued that the voice has more often been tuned to the advancement of the cause of family practice than to statesmanlike support of the health of the public. But the fact remains that the voice has produced a remarkable turnabout in the fortunes of these generalists in the last 25 years. And it is necessary to take into account this remarkable resurgence if one is to understand the contrapuntal rise during those years of the American Society of Internal Medicine.

fresh out of medical school, wending his weary way around hospital wards in pursuit of new knowledge. Somebody proposed resolving the intern-internist confusion by adding a syllable, but "internalist" was awkward and somehow failed to evoke a clearer image in the listener's mind.

Practicing internists had trouble finding effective, short ways of describing their specialty. "Diagnostician" did stimulate a spark of recognition in some listeners but clearly failed to convey the increasingly important part that therapy and continuing care played in the internist's relationship with patients. Some internists settled for negative definitions: "I don't do surgery or deliver babies or take care of infants." Another option—"specialist in adult medicine"—triggered sort of a connection in some people, since most everybody knew what a pediatrician was, but it was a mouthful to say. Still other internists opted for explication by etymology: "I am a specialist in organs inside the body, like the heart, lungs, kidney, liver."

This approach was helpful, but an analytical listener might reason that the internist was responsible for everything not in the dermatologist's domain; in addition, the clear thinking analyst might be puzzled by the observation that obstetrician-gynecologists also dealt with organs inside the body cavity (if the listener was a woman, she might well remember what an "internal" exam was), that surgeons removed appendixes from the abdominal cavity, and that urologists also paid attention to kidneys.

Despite these semantic difficulties, internists gradually came to be recognized as a worthy replacement for the generalist, somebody meriting the right to be called special. Word got around about a difference in this kind of doctor's approach to care. First of all, he made appointments according to a schedule, so that patients did not have to wait for hours in a crowded waiting room. Second, he did thorough evaluations, taking an hour to complete and including a host of questions about one's symptoms, medical history, personal and family history, and winding up with a complete stem-to-stern physical examination. Sometimes he would arrange for laboratory tests or x-rays or electrocardiograms. Third, on routine office visits, whether for some acute illness or for follow-up of a chronic problem, he would set aside enough time (sometimes 30 minutes!) to deal with it thoroughly. Finally, and perhaps most important, he took the time to get to know his patients personally so that he could deal with them as human beings, people with fears and feelings and families. Yet with all this, he was clearly highly competent, solving intricate medical problems as they arose and handling hospital care with efficiency and effectiveness.

One other element distinguished the internist from the general practitioner: the internist's fees tended to be higher. Not that individual patients objected; that thorough stem-to-stern appraisal was often the first time he or she had ever had a comprehensive history and physical exam and it was worth the 25 dollars for the hour it took. And the five-dollar fee for the 15 to 30 minute office visit for an acute illness or follow-up care was certainly a bargain compared to the three dollars charged by the GP for a few hurried minutes of time.

But if patients were willing to pay internists' charges with few qualms, the same was not true for third parties. Health insurance managers lived in a simple world in which an office visit was an office visit, no matter how long it took or what the qualifications were of the physician providing it. The managers would listen to reason if they could be pinned down firmly enough, but they couldn't change fee schedules without the approval of their boards of directors—which were often dominated by GPs and surgeons. Anyhow, it was hard to understand this new generalist role of the internist; he used to be a pure consultant—and "consultation" was a service health insurers could easily understand and pay for.

The solution for internists, obviously, was to educate the insurers about what internists actually do. The California Society of Internal Medicine's (CSIM's) major early accomplishment was to persuade insurers, especially California's Blue Shield plan, to adopt a schedule which included those services characteristic of the practice of internal medicine (and to qualify for such special payments, it was almost essential that the physician become a member of CSIM).

While single battles like CSIM's with Blue Shield were won from time to time, the war as a whole could not be won without an overall strategy for describing the entire range of physicians' services and for providing a device for relating one service to another. Again, Californians took the lead, this time with CSIM members in the forefront of the effort. In 1956, the California Medical Association (CMA) produced the first Relative Value Scale, in which the gamut of physician procedures was laid out in detail and—the astonishing result of countless hours of committee work—their relative worth to one another identified by unit numbers. Years later (until the FTC stepped in and called the RVS a fee-setting conspiracy) this innovative work would have widespread national acceptance; one of its grandchildren would be the AMA's effort, a document called Current Procedural Terminology, much-shaped by ASIM influence.

What were the professional loyalties of internists in mid-century? With rare exception, internists starting practice automatically joined the AMA/state medical association/county medical society hierarchy. And CSIM and other fledgling internists' societies were careful to do their work under the umbrella of state and local medical societies.

But internists had another rite-of-passage to take. It was perhaps even more automatic to "take the Board"—pass the written and oral examinations of the American Board of Internal Medicine—and then to seek membership, first as a member, later as a full Fellow, of the American College of Physicians.

The Board had, by 1956, certified more than 12,000 internists. These Diplomates automatically acquired a certain status, at least in the eyes of their colleagues. Perhaps they also achieved a more easy ascent through the levels of hospital medical staffs. But, "being Boarded" meant little to patients (unless while waiting, they read the handsome certificate mounted on the examining room wall), and it meant nothing as far as getting paid was concerned.

The ACP, founded in 1915, had more than 9,000 members in 1956, of whom two-thirds were Fellows. It was not a pure culture of internists, "internal medicine" having been interpreted broadly so as to let in a sprinkling of other non-surgeons, including some pathologists, radiologists, dermatologists, neurologists, and psychiatrists. (Its counterpart, the American College of Surgeons, is also an umbrella organization for all specialists performing surgery; the difference for surgeons is that individual surgical specialists—urologists, neurosurgeons, orthopedists, etc.—also have separate specialty boards and strong separate colleges or academies to serve them.)

But the ACP was and is primarily an organization of internists, and its principal mission has always been to further the education of its members and the profession generally. These functions were carried out primarily through its journal, *Annals of Internal Medicine*, its annual meeting, its regional programs and postgraduate courses. Although its membership was made up of practicing physicians, its leadership—the ones responsible for mounting the ACP educational thrust—was heavily weighted with academic internists from the nation's medical schools.

The College in 1956 was a major force in the lives of internists all over the country, even though it was structured as a national organization and did not have state or local chapters. A major question arose for those internists who perceived the need to take collective action about economic issues: should the College be the vehicle for organizing and coordinating that action?

Certainly, there was evidence of interest in the subject among the College's leadership. One of its Regents was Dwight Wilbur who had participated with fellow San Franciscans in getting CSIM started some ten years earlier. Another College leader interested in economic issues was its Secretary General, Wallace Yater of Washington, DC, whom many expected to reach the top in both organizations but whose role was limited by his inability to travel by air. Dr. Yater did serve the College as Governor, Regent, and Secretary General for many years, and exerted a great influence on the then-new and growing ASIM. A College Governor, Elbert L. Persons, of Duke University, had helped organize the North Carolina SIM, and another Southern California Governor, Philip Corr, had been active in the CSIM venture.

The ACP had even appointed a committee in 1955, charged with studying the problem of prepaid health insurance. Its members had talked about the possibility of promoting activities on the state level through the offices of the Governors, but in April 1956, all remained at the discussion level.

One other route for expressing the professional loyalties of at least some internists was just beginning to appear on the scene about this time. The urge to specialize—partly caused by patient demand and partly by physician desire to pursue excellence—was so strong that the broad specialty of internal medicine found itself subdivided into subspecialty fields. In certain locales internists who called themselves cardiologists or gastroenterologists, for instance, were limiting their practices to a narrow discipline. Interestingly, their practices resembled the old consultant/diagnostician role of yore, in that they cared for many patients referred by other internists whose knowledge was more general. However, while most of these subspecialists took care of their own patients' general medical needs, as well as their highly specialized ones, they did not completely identify themselves as internists. The handwriting was on the wall: sooner or later these narrow specialists (some called them "super" specialists, but those caring about the primacy of the broad discipline of internal medicine preferred the prefix "sub") would inevitably seek their own journals, their own meetings, their own societies, and their own certification mechanism.

Thus, if internal medicine was in competition on one side for the generalist function with GPs/FPs, it was also soon to be in competition with its own component parts. These two, somewhat opposing, trends making up the identity crisis of internal medicine would be of continuing concern to the field for years to come.

The fact is that practicing internists, despite these multiple loyalties and allegiances, did not have a separate organizational focus dedicated to dealing with their identity crisis. The AMA/state association/county society hierarchical organizations were often dominated by GPs and surgeons. Even had this not been the case, these organizations would have to preserve their umbrella role and deal with the collective and multiple problems of all physicians, not just the unique problems of any one specialty. At the other pole, the subspecialty organizations were just getting under way, were involved with their own identity crisis, and, in any event, were universally focused on bioscientific and educational activities.

In the middle was the American College of Physicians, devoted primarily to the welfare of internists and internal medicine. Its purposes, as stated in its constitution, are: a) maintaining and advancing the highest possible standards of medical education, medical practice and medical research; and b) perpetuating the history and best traditions of medicine and medical ethics, maintaining both the dignity and efficiency of internal medicine in its relationship to public welfare.

Monday morning internist quarterbacks, looking back 25 years, can argue endlessly about whether or not the College could have successfully played the game that ASIM ended up in. The lack of discrete state organizations would have hindered the College in any game plan. And its top-down power structure tended to leave policy-making in the hands of the few, and those few came primarily from the academic world, not the world of patient care. The truth is that the College's leadership did not *want* to take on a struggle in social, political—and especially economic—arenas. This position may have been reached partly through timidity, a lack of confidence in the leadership's ability to cope with the new forces at work. Or it may have been assumed partly out of the loftiest of motives, the conviction that the profession should be above crass concerns about money and should continue to devote itself to bioscience and education.

Still, a real need existed for some sort of an organization to serve the collective interest of internists and their patients. A vacuum existed. Who—or what—would try to fill it?

3

The Predecessor Organizations
Avant-Garde Ancestors

In the middle third of this century, as the number of practicing internists grew and as their role in delivering medical care expanded, an interesting dispersion took place in the location of their practices—centrifugally, from their traditional concentration around major metropolitan teaching centers, to new settings in smaller cities, large towns, and suburbs.

In these new geographic circumstances, individual internists found some difficulties in keeping in touch with what was going on in their specialty. Apparently, collegial needs could not be solved simply by passing the Boards and getting elected to the College, nor by local hospital medical staff relationships. A new phenomenon arose, primarily springing up as internists settled down to practice after World War II, but sometimes appearing as early as the Depression years: internists banded together to establish an "academy" or "society" of internal medicine.

Some of these were in cities (Seattle, Brooklyn, Chicago, Salt Lake City had early ones), some at the county level (Saint Joseph, Indiana, and Westchester, New York, were organized in the early fifties), a few were regional (Western New York in 1952), and many were state-wide (California of course, but also Arizona, Oregon, Washington, Connecticut, and North Carolina, among others); there were academies in some Canadian provinces, and there was talk of extending the west coast groups across the ocean to Hawaii in what could have been the Pan-Pacific Society of Internal Medicine.

These developing organizations shared certain characteristics. One of their aims was simple conviviality, the chance to meet with one's colleagues in a spirit of good fellowship and to chat about mutual interests. Another was to provide, for shared benefit, programs of continuing medical education.

It would not be unusual if internists thus gathered together, having had their fill of gastronomic and intellectual fare, might turn to consideration of economic needs. In fact, it would have been surprising if they, with their problem-solving aptitudes, had failed to consider the difficulty in getting appropriate reimbursement from third parties. Nor would it be unlikely that internists, meeting for other purposes, might still find time to discuss their identity, their role in the scheme of things, and their differences from other practitioners.

The credit for the first major structural organization, one principally devoted to grappling with the economic and managerial aspects of internists' practices, goes without question to the Californians. It may be that their pioneer spirit made them more ready and willing than their Eastern colleagues to do battle with the incursions of bureaucratic third parties, or perhaps it was because they were simply the first to be exposed to the new set of problems. California was the place where health insurance started and the first place where third parties became a major source of payments to physicians for their services. Whatever their incentive, the Californians took the lead in addressing the new circumstances and dealing with them successfully.

The California Society had its origins in San Francisco just after the end of World War II. In that city, Dwight Wilbur (whose medical statesmanship would later be recognized in his becoming the president of the ACP in 1959, the president of AMA in 1968-69—and ASIM's first Distinguished Internist in 1969) and a number of practicing colleagues—Walter Beckh, William Bender, Ed Bruck, DeWitt T. Burnham, Allen Hinman, and others—met and established an informal group to study the economic problems of the internist. Thereafter (as Burnham later described it at the ASIM Founders Meeting), "telephones got hot and groups were formed in Los Angeles, San Diego, Santa Barbara, Fresno, Stockton and Sacramento." In 1946 representative groups of leading internists from various parts of California met concurrently with a meeting of the California Medical Association and formed CSIM.

How did the new CSIM go about the process of addressing the problems facing internal medicine in California? As described later at some length by Lewis Bullock at the Founders Meeting, it was an orderly and coordinated process—not unlike the internist's disciplined approach to solving a patient's problem.

The first task, accomplished particularly through the speeches of some of its presidents, was to set standards for the practice of internal medicine, specifying its scope and limits. The second task was to develop a system through which health insurers could reimburse properly for services characteristic of internal medicine; a schedule was created which defined office visit at different levels, through use of a separately identified listing of fees for internal medicine.

Apparently, negotiators for California's Blue Shield and Blue Cross were surprised to be confronted by a group with such a well worked-out program, and found it easy to go along with CSIM proposals. It was this strategy—having a reasonable, practical, workable program spelled out—that, combined with membership unity and a developing public relations program, made CSIM a force to be reckoned with.

There was no doubt in Bullock's mind that these strategies were successful. His summation of CSIM accomplishments to the Founders Meeting is a proud one: "This society, by defining internal medicine, insisting on high standards, letting the profession and the public know how its members practice, has tremendously improved the economic status of the internist."

Imbued with evangelical fervor, the Californians, while conscientiously concentrating on their work at home, had energy left over to help out internists elsewhere. Perceiving that the problems confronting internists in California existed in other states, yet detecting no parallel strong organizational thrusts anywhere else, CSIM, in 1952, appointed an Interstate Coordinating Committee, under the chairmanship of San Francisco internist Walter Beckh. Ten other Western states were invited to meet with CSIM during its 1952 annual meeting in Santa Barbara.

As a direct result of the discussions there, Arizona soon formed its own statewide society (perhaps stimulated by an Arizona Blue Shield proposal to add nonsurgical hospital care to its schedule). Oregon and Washington followed suit, but other states, whether from small size, timidity, or lack of leadership, failed to suit up for the game. (Nevada thought for a time that merger with its large and effective neighbor to the west would best serve its needs.)

Nonetheless, the internist grapevine carried the news in all directions. Beckh received letters expressing interest from internists in many other states, some citing individual personal concerns, others expressing the collective interest of their established local academies and societies of internal medicine.

By the end of 1955, the threads of enthusiasm had been spun and the Californians were eager to see if they—although scattered—could be woven into a tapestry of national scope. At its January 1956 meeting, the CSIM council unanimously passed a resolution proposing the formation of a national organization. Dr. Beckh, as chairman of the Interstate Coordinating Committee, was charged with issuing invitations to internist organizations throughout North America. (He prepared the invitation list with great care, inviting primarily clinicians who were in their forties, were members of the ACP, were certified by the ABIM, and whom he thought would be likely to attend the Los Angeles meeting.)

Dr. Beckh's letter, written on CSIM stationery and dated March 9, 1956, is a classic instance of the internist's use of an orderly presentation of data. The first paragraph states the why of the founding ten years earlier of CSIM ("the unusual growth of voluntary health insurance in California"). The second paragraph asserts that "the same problem has become countrywide" and that "more than merely local and state organizations are needed to present our point of view." The paragraph ends with the announcement that the CSIM council had "passed a motion to consider plans for the formation of an American Society of Internal Medicine."

The third paragraph extends the invitation to attend and lays out the circumstances of the meeting. "(It) is scheduled to be held Sunday, April 15 at 10:30 a.m. . . . This meeting will certainly last past the lunch hour and well into the afternoon, so that the persons attending it should not make plans for other engagements before 5:00 p.m." The last paragraph winds matters up and adds just a touch of weightiness: "Our organization feels that this scheduled meeting is a most important and crucial one for internal medicine in America. We hope most urgently that you or an officially delegated representative of your society will be able to attend it."

The Californians had done all that had to be done to get the birthing of ASIM under way. They could still make detailed preparations to insure that the fateful April meeting would be conducted in an orderly and informative fashion. But in the end it would be up to others, the non-California attendees, to decide if the aspiration of California would be translated into a nationwide dream on behalf of internists and their patients.

4

The Founders Meeting

Auspicious Atmosphere

Dr. Beckh's letter of invitation produced an astonishing turnout. To be sure, of the forty-one men attending the opening session, thirteen were from California—Beckh, Bullock, Burnham, Callaway, Corr, Davis, Hoagland, Martin, Mumler, Rumsey, Steeley, Thompson, and George Wever of Stockton, who chaired the meeting. But there were many attendees who had traveled long distances, partly for this meeting, partly to attend the annual ACP sessions starting the next day. Two were Canadians, from Alberta (Balfour) and British Columbia (Hertzman). East Coast states were well represented: Seigle from Connecticut, Baganz from Delaware, Yater from Washington D.C., Clark from New York, Gilmour (and Persons who was his state's official representative but busy at College Governor affairs) from North Carolina, and Wilson from South Carolina.

Other Eastern states also sent representatives: Kentucky (Llewellyn), Tennessee (Chaney). Mid-Western states likewise sent individual physicians: Indiana (Grorud), Ohio (Goudsmit), Missouri (Farris), Michigan (Taylor), Wisconsin (Gilbert). Minnesota managed to be represented by three attendees (Fuller, Greenberg, and Schaaf). Naturally, the Western states were well represented: Arizona (Bank, Fair), Colorado (Livingston), Idaho (Call, Howard, Johnson), New Mexico (January), Oregon (Boylston, Maurice), Utah (Orme, Wilkinson), Washington (Goss). And even the Territory of Hawaii had its own representative (Johnson).

The program moved along with symphonic precision, its orchestration reflecting prior planning by the Californians, the conductor being the CSIM president George Wever. The first movement belonged exclusively to the California group: DeWitt Burnham related the history of the founding of the CSIM. Lewis Bullock described the what and how of CSIM accomplishments to date with special reference to prepaid health insurance involving "third parties." Paul Hoagland detailed its public relations program (including an article about internists, authored by Paul DeKruif and appearing in *The Reader's Digest*). Walter Beckh reported his efforts to get other North American internist groups to follow CSIM's lead. James Thompson presented data about Blue

Shield's national accounts. Claude Callaway spoke up for internal medicine having a "loud voice" at the local, state and national levels. He also hoped that all internists would understand the position of the College, and one of its Governors, Philip Corr, reported that many College Regents "are favorably disposed to an organization such as this."

The floor was now thrown open for non-Californians to present their views. Honolulu's Elmer Johnson reported that Hawaii's internists were ready to address economic issues. Ernest Wilkinson of Salt Lake City related problems with insurers in Utah, and B. F. Fuller cited similar difficulties in Minnesota. Kent Thayer of Phoenix asked "how do you define an internist?," and got an excellent in-depth response from Lewis Bullock, who listed such attributes as training, certification, performance with patients, recordkeeping, desire to stay informed, and above all, interest in the patient as a whole. Seattle's Clark Goss expressed concerns about criteria for membership in a new national society. Arnoldus Goudsmit of Youngstown, Ohio, also voiced worries about qualifications, to which Los Angeles' William Mumler replied that third party reimbursement should be based on two factors—time and ability—and not whether a physician was called an internist or a general practitioner.

Perhaps sensing a consensus developing, Wever asked Bullock to discuss the recently passed CSIM resolution proposing consideration of a national organization. Pointing out that internists nationally were at much the same point that Californians had been ten years earlier, Bullock offered the opinion that "We can not survive alone" and that nobody else could take the necessary steps. He then proceeded to offer the following resolution:

> "I would therefore move, Mr. Chairman, that this group go on record as forming an American Society of Internal Medicine; that the members of this group constitute the original forming body of such an organization; that the members here go back to their respective organizations and present such a proposal and that another meeting of this group be held at a convenient time to formulate and define the Society; that the Chairman appoint a committee in the meantime to draw up articles of incorporation and bylaws and a nominating committee, to make this a functioning, effective national organization with invitations to all of the states to form similar bodies to become partners in the American Society."

The motion was seconded by Dr. Goss of Seattle.

Wever carefully allowed time for discussion of the motion. Robert Gilbert said that the newly formed Wisconsin SIM would favor a national organization. Hartford's Stewart Seigle said that Connecticut's year-old SIM was in favor of a national organization, but felt "it should be a federation, rather than a strong central national organization." Comments were offered about the purposes of the new organization (should it be interested in economics, or just the quality of practice?) and about its organizational structure.

At this juncture Wever decided it was time to call for a vote "upon the motion that you have heard initiating the formation of the American Society of Internal Medicine. All those in favor were asked to signify by saying 'aye.'"

The motion was passed unanimously.

"Very well," Wever said, "we will assume that this group will be the founding group."

The first session still wasn't quite over. Ways and means of getting the show on the road were discussed. It was agreed that a steering committee would be appointed to advance the cause.

Wever advised that the College had extended an invitation to make a presentation before the combined meeting of the Regents and Governors that afternoon. It was agreed that the Wever-Bullock-Beckh team would represent the group well. It was further agreed that the founding group should meet again—at 3:30 p.m.—to learn of the College's reaction and to discuss further plans.

Wever called the afternoon session to order at 3:45 p.m. This time there was an overflow crowd, much the same group as for the morning session plus other internists who had heard about the excitement.

The chairman reported that Lewis Bullock had presented the gist of the morning's deliberations to a combined meeting of the College's Boards of Regents and Governors with great skill and in a highly diplomatic manner. The result had been most reassuring. The combined Boards had already decided that "they were in accord with the movement of the California Society in furthering the cause of the economic status of the internist . . . and that they did not choose to participate in the program."

The endorsement of the College thus safely in hand, Wever proceeded to announce the appointment of a steering committee for the founding group with Bullock as chairman, Callaway as secretary, and as members Paul Clark of Syracuse, Fuller of Minnesota, Gilbert of Wisconsin, Goss of Washington State, Victor Hertzman of Vancouver, Johnson of Hawaii, John Llewellyn of Louisville, Seigle of Connecticut, and Wilkinson of New Mexico (subsequently, N. Litton January of Albuquerque and Elbert Persons of Durham were added.)

The chair was then turned over to the new chairman, who promptly demonstrated his organizing ability, outlining certain problems facing the new organization such as staffing, equipment, personnel, and finances. He proposed using the existing facilities of the CSIM to satisfy temporarily the first three of those needs. He answered the fourth by offering a contribution or loan by CSIM of $1,500—at the same time expressing the hope that other societies would provide similar support to the new ASIM.

The discussion then turned to other items needing consideration in the first months of the new Society's life. Agreement was reached about the fact that there should be some kind of dues structure, but not about its amount ($2, $3, or $5?). Arrangements were made to receive money (Callaway was given the job of treasurer as well as secretary), to work out a draft Constitution and Bylaws (Goss, Gilbert and Seigle were charged with the task), and to have a Nominating Committee. Most formalities could be finalized a year later at the new Society's first Annual Meeting in Boston, but in the interim the Steering Committee would serve as the temporary governing body and its chairman as the president pro tem.

The shape of the inchoate organization having thus been sketched in, the Bylaws Committee was charged with fleshing in some details for consideration by the founders several days later. The meeting ajourned at 5 p.m.

Dr. Bullock called to order the final session of the founding group at 5:30 p.m. on Wednesday, April 18, 1956. The Society had been unable to obtain a large room for the meeting, so that many attendees listened and participated from the foyer and hall. (One such was Clyde Greene, who, while present and actively involved in ASIM affairs for years thereafter, inadvertently found his name left off the roster of the founding group.)

The principal order of business was to discuss the draft Constitution and Bylaws presented by the committee's chairman, Clark Goss. The content was straightforward enough, detailing in 14 articles provisions for the name, location, objectives, membership, council, executive committee, officers, meetings, committees, dues, penalties, amendments, dissolution and parliamentary procedure. But the specific sections under the important articles were discussed in detail, with many revisions proposed and ultimately accepted. Nearly four hours had passed by the time it was finally "moved, seconded, and carried unanimously that they are to be further studied by the component societies and finally presented for adoption at the next meeting of the group." The meeting adjourned at 9:15 p.m.

ASIM was in business.

5

Intraprofessional Relationships
Anxious Attachments

Surfing connoisseurs tell us that most waves are imperfect; some crest too high, too early and disappear shortly; others have a long run, but are shallow and without force. Only a few are just right, peaking early yet with enough internal energy to give a sustained run. ASIM seems to have come close to achieving that perfect form in its first five years, its sustained power provided by its early leaders.

Or, perhaps, ASIM's astonishing early vigor came not from a few energetic leaders but from the fact that the environmental conditions, specifically the needs of practicing internists, were just right. A different, probably more apt, metaphor was offered by ASIM's first president, Lewis Bullock, whose description of the Society's early support by internists was "like dropping a crystal into a super-saturated solution."

Whatever figure of speech one prefers, the evidence is clear that, from its inception, ASIM was an alert, bustling, vigilant organization. And it is equally plain that nearly all of the problems that the early leaders had to face were ones that would pop up again and again like boardwalk shooting targets over the next two decades or so.

Like all fledglings, the ASIM baby was impelled to call itself to the attention of other bodies in its arena of activity. It is not clear if the selection of one or the other of two principal strategies—make friends or pick a fight—was made in each instance by purposeful design, but it is certain that both methods were used.

In the case of the 1956 American College of Surgeons (ACS) brouhaha, the chip-on-the-shoulder option was taken. On November 16, 1956, Dr. Bullock, as chairman of the interim committee, sent a "MEMORANDUM TO ALL STATE SOCIETIES" quoting a report printed in California newspapers of a statement by Paul R. Hawley, then the director of the ACS, "that nearly half of the Blue Shield plans throughout the country are guilty of unethical fee splitting because, without raising insurance premiums or fees paid, they have deprived surgeons of their fair share of income by paying part of it to the internist or general practitioner who sees the patient before or after the operation." Bullock had already fired off a letter to ACS Regents' chairman I. S. Ravdin asking for verification and explanation of the statement.

Ravdin and Hawley both replied, denying any attempt on the part of ACS to denigrate internists; Hawley's statement not only denied having said that "internists were receiving an improper portion of the fees from various insurance companies," he also affirmed his opinion that qualified internists were the most underpaid of any specialty in medicine.

Bullock had gotten a decisive and satisfying reply to his query—and, incidentally, had found a tidy little way of demonstrating, to existing and potential ASIM constituencies, the new organization's clout.

A somewhat similar controversy, this time with the shoe on the other foot, took place in late 1957. A pamphlet had been received by certain citizens of Melrose, Massachusetts, praising specialists and vilifying general practitioners—"(their) black bag has now become a symbol . . . of inadequate medical care." When Dr. Jack DeTar, president of the American Academy of General Practice, complained to Chairman Bullock, that energetic person promptly investigated (through Frank Christopher, secretary-treasurer of the Massachusetts SIM), and finding no evidence of internist culpability, wrote a soothing letter to Dr. DeTar who, in reply, expressed his expectation of continued cooperation between the two organizations. Naturally, copies of the correspondence were quickly dispatched to all state societies of internal medicine.

Incidentally, as part of the correspondence, Dr. DeTar had expressed concern about ASIM's (mostly Dr. Bullock's) use of the phrase "family physician" to describe a part of an internist's work. Obviously, the AAGP was beginning to entertain the notion of changing itself into the AAFP.

Friendly relationships with the AMA, deemed by Society leaders then as now to be a desirable goal, were pursued assiduously. In January 1958, the ASIM position was codified: ASIM was largely in accord with the AMA and would ordinarily cooperate with the AMA, but would "continue to present problems directly to the Congress and to direct the component societies to continue to contact their Congressmen where indicated." The motion, unanimously carried, set out a policy that still obtains.

The Society's first official dealings with the AMA came after what Clark Goss described as "insistent communications . . . (with) the Council on Medical Service of the AMA." He, as chairman of ASIM's Medical Services Committee, and President Bullock were invited to appear at a meeting of the Council's Subcommittee on Prepayment Medical Care Plans on August 10, 1957. Dr. Goss' written report (sent to all ASIM members—then numbering about 4,000) contained this marvelous paragraph:

> "The weather being something less than pleasant in Chicago, the AMA Committee's two day meeting was held at a not readily accessible recreation area 80 miles west of Port Angeles, Washington. Accordingly, Dr. Bullock flew from Los Angeles to Seattle Friday night, August 9; together, we made our way to the meeting Saturday a.m. where, immediately upon our arrival, we were very courteously received by the Committee, so that after a two hour session, we were able to return to Seattle from whence Dr. Bullock flew home that same night; he is now known to me as 'Iron Man Bullock.'"

Dr. Goss comments on Bullock's approach to the subcommittee: "With his facility of speaking, choice of words, and well-turned phrases and complete grasp of our problems, Dr. Bullock gave an excellent presentation to the committee." Such clarity was apparently necessary, since "those present seemed unaware that . . . internist services are not adequately provided for . . . in most prepayment plan fee schedules." Bullock and Goss went on to educate subcommittee members about what an internist is (no longer just a consultant) and what he does. "Dr. Bullock and I both emphasized the matters of *time* involved in the complete history and physical examination and the *cost* in carrying on a practice of internal medicine because of the number of employees required, office space required, etc."

Happily, the educational briefing bore fruit. A December 1957 report to the AMA House of Delegates by the AMA Council on Medical Service cited its belief in "the possibility that physicians, in their way, are just as skillful as the surgeons in their way, and they should be recompensed accordingly." Among the Council's three recommendations was this one: "that the House of Delegates endorse the idea of the development by this committee of a relative value schedule of medical and surgical services and at the present moment suggest the California scale as a good example, because of its specific reference to the values of diagnostic and medical services, as well as surgical services."

But the wheels of the AMA sometimes grind slowly—and not infrequently need further external push. Frustrated by delays, the ASIM House of Delegates, at the Annual Meeting in Miami in May 1961, finally approved the presentation of a formal resolution to the AMA:

Subject: "Descriptive Coding of Medical Services

> "WHEREAS, there is an increasing utilization of and therefore need for detailed descriptive listings and coding of the services offered in medical care, and
> "WHEREAS, these descriptive codings must therefore be established in sufficient detail that all areas of medical service are fairly and properly defined, and
> "WHEREAS, to date, there has been inadequate descriptive

> coding of the varied and numerous nonsurgical services of medical care, and
> "WHEREAS, a persisting lack of adequate descriptive coding of nonsurgical services of medical care will exclude these services and therefore cause a deterioration in the quality and availability of medical care, THEREFORE, BE IT
> "RESOLVED that the American Medical Association immediately initiate the study and development of more adequate and detailed descriptive coding of services of medical care and, BE IT FURTHER
> "RESOLVED, that the American Medical Association shall establish a means of continuing study for improving the detailed descriptive codings of all medical care so that new procedures may be quickly incorporated into all schedules which depend on such descriptive coding for the supplying or reimbursement of costs of medical care."

On June 28, 1961, Carter Smith of Georgia, delegate to the AMA and a future Board member of ASIM, presented the resolution to the AMA House. After some discussion, the reference committee commented favorably: "Resolution 83 calls attention to an obvious weakness in most of the prepayment insurance schedules and many of the relative value study listings of services. This weakness is a lack of adequate descriptive coding of nonsurgical services."

The resolution was unanimously approved by the House—nearly four years after ASIM's presentation to the subcommittee.

It can be argued that the climate was ripe for the AMA to come to this position anyhow. The California RVS was receiving considerable attention and the desirability of uniform nomenclature and coding of medical care services was being recognized—especially since Blue Shield and others were developing their own systems. But ASIM's pressure was surely a significant force in persuading the AMA to take on descriptive coding as one of its projects. This 1961 resolution started the effort that has produced, over a nearly 20-year span, four editions of *Current Procedural Terminology.* Within the text of that constantly evolving handbook is a section—largely shaped by key ASIM participants—that describes in considerable detail the services of the internist.

One intraprofessional relationship of the early years that seemingly needed no special effort to keep harmonious (but naturally got such an effort anyway) was that with the American College of Physicians. After all, ASIM was born with the College's blessing and it could be said that the College assisted—as a behind-the-scenes accessory—before, during, and immediately after the birthing. The Regents endorsed ASIM's creation and its executive secretary, Ed Loveland, sent a baptismal declaration of the Regents' approval by formal letter. The mutual spirit of harmony and cooperation was highly visible during ASIM's early years, with virtually no hint of troubled times ahead.

The CSIM newsletter of May 28, 1956, announcing the process and outcome of the founding meeting, put the early mood well: "At the present time it would appear that the American College of Physicians will continue its traditional aims of furthering the educational and academic goal of medicine in this country and it would seem that they are not prepared nor desire to undertake activity in an economic field. The Founding Members of the American Society of Internal Medicine therefore consider their activities to be entirely appropriate and complementary to the activities of the American College of Physicians and do not consider that the proposed group will be in any sense in competition with the College."

The earliest version of ASIM Bylaws specified that the annual meeting of the ASIM Council (later Board of Trustees) should take place at the same time and place as the annual meeting of the ACP. Article 3 Section 4 stated that a purpose of ASIM was "to complement and supplement the aims and activities of the ACP." Article 4 Section 3 stated that one of the qualifications for membership in ASIM was membership in ACP. An eight-page pamphlet, listing the purposes of ASIM and published in October of 1957 (one could get extra copies at 19¢ a pamphlet), devoted much of the first page to the ASIM-ACP relationship: "Though independent of the American College of Physicians, this organization has been recognized by that body as the economic spokesman for the medical specialists of our states and in our nation. Established committees provide liaison between these two bodies whose common aim is to secure the finest medical care by means of the educational and scientific programs of the American College of Physicians in a secure economic position made possible by the program of the American Society of Internal Medicine."

At the second annual ASIM meeting in Atlantic City in April 1958, Wallace Yater, secretary general of ACP and member of the Executive Committee of ASIM, reported on the smooth relationship: "ASIM, in establishing definite purposes and criteria for membership, has received active support from the ACP." He closed "with the recommendation that every state have a strong SIM with all qualified internists as members."

At that same meeting, Stewart Seigle, chairman of ASIM's Public Relations Committee, announced that ACP would be asked to reserve a section in its publication *The Annals of Internal Medicine* for news of ASIM. This request was granted for a while.

In 1957 the Board of Regents established an ACP Liaison Committee which would meet with the Executive Committee of ASIM. In 1958 Dr. Robert Wilson, chairman of the Liaison Committee, received a report that ASIM was well satisfied with the publication of its news in the *Annals*. At that meeting, it was agreed that liaison between the two organizations should be encouraged at a state level and "that regional meetings be integrated whenever possible."

In 1958, and for some years thereafter, ASIM had booths in the scientific exhibit rooms for the annual meetings of both ACP and AMA. (At one such, the ASIM member in charge of the booth fell ill and his place was taken by a rotating group of hastily trained local ASIM wives.)

A May 1958 special article in the *New England Journal of Medicine* by Chester S. Keefer, MD, professor of medicine at Boston University, presented in scholarly fashion a justification for ASIM's existence and a rationale for a continued separation-of-power status between the College and the Society. He prophesied (with remarkable prescience) that " in the future the Society might well have papers read by men who are experts in the field of medical economics, social security, medical insurance, hospital insurance, and so forth. . ."

An early sixties issue of *The Bulletin,* begun in 1960 to give a bimonthly account of ACP affairs, featured an article by the newly elected president of ASIM, Ross Taylor. Entitled "The American College of Physicians and the American Society of Internal Medicine," the paper reviewed the history of ASIM's birth and of ACP's involvement in, and reaction to that event. It concluded: "The relationships between the American College of Physicians and the American Society of Internal Medicine since the founding of the Society have remained close and cordial. The view of the writer, expressed several times in the past, is that there is one great body of internists dedicated to maintaining and improving standards of patient care, and accomplishing this with one hand, through the American College of Physicians and its continuing educational facilities and requirements for advancement; and also with another hand, through the American Society of Internal Medicine with its component societies with their constant requirements as to standards of practice and with the recognition and development of solutions to socioeconomic problems which affect the patient or the internist. It would seem essential that all internists be active members of both organizations."

In the beginning, ASIM efforts to relate to other groups were not very discriminating. Early presidents and other officers were kept busy scurrying around the country trying to increase the visibility of the young organization by attending meetings of all kinds and descriptions. An introduction from the dais at meetings of the American Hospital Association, the Association of American Medical Colleges, the Southern Medical Association, and others, could not help but further the Society's prestige.

Gradually, however, it became apparent that such random travels were exhausting, both for individuals and the budget. Rough criteria—a foreshadow of one of ASIM's guiding principles in the 1970s—were established to weigh a proposed visit's or project's cost against its potential effectiveness in achieving present objectives. ASIM's major emphasis on economics and on the internist's role led it to concentrate in the beginning on other bodies with shared or overlapping interests: The College of American Pathologists, The American College of Radiology, The American Academy of General Practice, and the American Academy of Pediatrics. Such liaisons continue to this day.

6

Insurers and Government
Artful Associations

ASIM's early efforts to establish productive relationships with other organizations were not limited to professional groups within organized medicine. A different kind of relationship was sought—and, with some difficulty, achieved—with associations representing health insurers (which were just beginning to be called "third-party payors").

Looking back from the eighties, we tend to think that governmental incursions into the practice of internal medicine didn't begin until the dramatic Medicare-Medicaid legislation of the mid-sixties. The fact is that ASIM's earliest activities on behalf of its members (and its potential members) involved a government program—and there was no dearth of similar problems during its early years.

Early attention was paid to the private (sometimes inappropriately called "commercial") health insurers through their collective organizations, the Health Insurance Association of America (HIAA) and the Health Insurance Council (HIC). Clark Goss, in 1957 chairman of ASIM's Medical Services Committee (and later the Society's fourth president), wrote to the associate director for health insurance of the HIAA, outlining ASIM's position that "health insurance programs, by and large, have ignored the specialty of internal medicine and the traditional and necessary position of the internist in the medical community." He went on to say, "We look with favor upon health insurance embodying major medical expense, catastrophic illness or dollar deductible coverage; here, it would seem, sound insurance principles could be applied."

Dr. Goss' position seems little short of prophetic, at least when viewed in light of subsequent ASIM policy. In any event, the record shows that HIAA promptly replied and an ongoing relationship was thereby established between ASIM and the private health insurers (one that later included semi-annual golf games between an ASIM Health Insurance Committee chairman and representatives—Paul Robinson and Al Larson—of the HIC). And one other benefit came of this exchange of correspondence—HIAA Associate Director, Albert V. Whitehall, three years later would become ASIM's second Executive Director.

A less expeditious outcome arose with ASIM's overtures to the other major segment of the private sector health insurers, the Blues, represented by the National Association of Blue Shield Plans (NABSP). The first official recognition of the existence of a problem between internists and Blue Shield carriers came during ASIM's second annual meeting in Atlantic City in April 1958. A resolution, presented by Washington, D.C. member William B. Walsh (a member of ASIM's Medical Services Committee, later the first chairman of its Legislative Committee, and, still later, founder of the Good Ship Hope and the Hope Foundation), was passed, pleading for all local Blue Shield plans to recognize the services of internists in their fee schedules and threatening that ASIM members might withdraw as participating physicians if the plans failed to do so.

But the Blues were not eager to accede to ASIM's request, arguing that change in the Blue Shield fee system would not be practical. Finally, in June 1961, officers and Trustees of ASIM met with top officials of NABSP in New York to discuss what kinds of fee schedules would be used by NABSP in its national accounts. According to an August 1961 ASIM newsletter, "It was agreed that small working committees would be appointed from each group to seek a practical and harmonious solution for the many problems which exist." ASIM representatives were James Feffer of Washington, D.C., Bowen Taylor of Omaha and Bert Bullington of Saginaw, Michigan.

The crux of the problem was that Blue Shield, cognizant of the growing enthusiasm for relative value schedules, had decided to devise its own system, the Professional Services Index, and the initial draft of the PSI failed to acknowledge the services of internal medicine.

The ASIM subcommittee, after some tough negotiations with their opposite numbers in Blue Shield, achieved all of its goals. As reported by President Taylor, "The negotiations resulted in the following procedures being definitely accepted for listing on the NABSP Professional Services Index: 1) routine medical care; 2) concurrent medical care; 3) intensive medical care; 4) consultations, both limited and complete, with these consultations to be available as specific items even though followed by continuing care of the patient on the part of the consultant; and 5) prolonged detention." NABSP also agreed to incorporate the specific item of "history and physical examination" as a hospital care benefit as soon as they incorporated it in outpatient codings.

While this triumph of ASIM negotiators applied only to national accounts and did not bind any of the many individual Blue Shield plans to use the new schedule in local marketing, it nonetheless exerted considerable pressure on those plans to conform, and assisted ASIM's component societies immeasurably in waging the battle locally.

Once the battle was over and internists' services were recognized in Blue Shield schedules, relationships between ASIM and NABSP became easy and mutually respectful. Future ASIM Health Insurance Committee chairmen would attend NABSP meetings as a matter of course, perhaps fuss about some aspect of the Blue Shield schedules (for instance, how does the internist report the subtle differences between "consultation" and "concurrent care?"), but major confrontations and negotiating battles were no longer needed.

In July 1956, the 84th Congress passed a bill called "Medicare"—nearly ten years before Medical Care for the Aged legislation earned that sobriquet for good—to provide payment for medical care for dependents of armed service personnel. The Department of Defense, administrators of the program, used a "modern" nomenclature modeled after the California Medical Associations's Relative Value Schedule, but inexplicably, omitted item 028—complete history and physical examination. Lewis Bullock, as chairman of ASIM's Interim Committee, strongly objected to the Department of Defense, and the Medicare problem was a major topic of discussion at ASIM's first Annual Meeting in Boston in April 1957.

Dr. Bullock was also promoting internal medicine's recognition in other federal health programs. The VA at that time had a Hometown Care Program, providing payment for services to veterans from private physicians. Again, the schedule failed to cover the history and physical exam service, and again, Dr. Bullock complained. The result was favorable—the VA agreed, at least for its California constituents, to insert the desired nomenclature in its schedule.

Dr. Bullock kept looking for—and finding—new causes around which to rally internists. In November 1957, he pointed out to the presidents of all state societies of internal medicine that the federal government was proposing a public assistance program for indigents in which the payment would be set at 80 percent of the normal Relative Value Schedule. The CSIM had adopted a resolution objecting to the proposal as "cut rate" medicine, and Bullock suggested that other state SIMs should pass similar resolutions for submission to their state medical societies.

The following January, Bullock sent a letter to the Chairman of the House Ways and Means Committee (yes, it was Wilbur Mills), announcing ASIM's opposition to the Forand bill which would have paid the cost of hospital, nursing home, and surgical services for OASI eligibles. The last paragraph deserves mention: "Please be aware of the great cost to the federal government if this legislation is enacted. Burdened as we already are with our tax load and facing the need for great expenditures for defense, surely you cannot favor adding another load."

The common denominator from ASIM's viewpoint in all of these legislative bits and pieces was the way medical services were listed in fee schedules. In January 1958, ASIM's Executive Committee "unanimously voted to urge all component state societies to request that the term 'special medical procedures' be changed in all future fee schedules to read 'section on internal medicine.'" Clark Goss followed up with a letter asking state SIMs to develop their own fee schedules and to submit them to ASIM for preparation of an average fee schedule. It is worthy of note that these recommendations were made without any worry about anti-trust action by the Federal Trade Commission.

At the Atlantic City Annual Meeting of the Society, William Walsh made a lengthy report to the House, including the observation that "in the last session of Congress over 400 bills bearing upon the sick, the treatment of the sick or some other phase of medicine were introduced."

On July 26, 1961, a major event in ASIM's brief history took place. President-Elect Stewart Seigle testified in person at the House Ways and Means Committee, opposing the Health Insurance Benefits Act of 1961 (that year's version of a Social Security program to pay for hospital and outpatient services for those over 65). Seigle's delivery was calm, the speech's content sound, and the arguments cogent. Apparently, it impressed the committee, one of whose members, Bruce Alger of Texas, took the unusual step of writing Dr. Seigle to congratulate him on "your splendid presentation." The bill, like similar ones before it, failed to make it out of committee, and it would continue to fail for four more years.

However, the involvement of government in medical care at the federal, and to a lesser degree at the state, level was increasing by leaps and bounds. Equally clearly, ASIM was finding it necessary to pay increasing attention to legislative matters. Characteristically, ASIM geared up to make legislation one of the high priority items on its extensive agenda of things to do.

7

Internal Affairs

Able Administration

Even fledgling organizations, if they are to conduct routine business, have to have resources—personnel, a headquarters office, and money. As might be expected, ASIM's early leaders paid suitable attention to these seemingly mundane, but necessary-for-survival matters.

The verbatim minutes of the Founders Meeting were recorded by CSIM's secretary, Mrs. Mildred Coleman, and she continued as ASIM's part-time secretary, courtesy of CSIM, for four years. An accomplished technician, she brought to her work a deep sense of involvement in her employer's activities. She never failed, no matter what the context, to spell internist with a capital I and internal medicine with a capital I and a capital M. (Interestingly, Fee Schedule also merited this distinction.) By the 1958 annual meeting, three other secretaries, Johanna Stracke, Dorothy Dodge and Shirley Purinton, were on hand to help with the transcribing chores. Shirley later was sent to Durham, North Carolina, to serve as secretary to ASIM's second president, Elbert Persons, working half-time for Duke University and half-time for ASIM.

As ASIM grew, the need for administrative expertise increased. In October 1958, the Society announced the appointment, effective January 1, 1959, of Mr. Robert L. Richards as ASIM's first executive secretary. Richards had worked in organized medicine since 1947 and since 1956 had been assistant director of the Pennsylvania Medical Society.

Two years later, Richards moved on to a new (and better-paid) executive job and G. Tod Bates was named as his acting successor (with Mrs. Stracke as executive assistant). A retired U.S. Air Force colonel, Bates had administrative know-how, if not much experience in the health field, as well as much talent and fame as a musician.

The search for a professional director with health care experience continued, and was finally concluded in August of 1961. Bates stayed on as associate director for four more years until his early and untimely death. The new exec was Albert V. Whitehall, already known to ASIM leaders as director of health insurance for the Life Insurance Association of America and as associate director of the HIAA. A native of Ontario and possessor of a law degree, Whitehall had worked in

Washington for the American Hospital Association and elsewhere for two Blue Cross plans. President Taylor announced the appointment, citing the new Executive Director's experience in "three sides of the health care field—hospitals, Blue Cross and insurance companies."

A growing organization needs a headquarters office. The Californian group found one for ASIM—small enough to be affordable, but large enough to hold secretarial staff and the burgeoning files—at 350 Post Street in the heart of San Francisco. This was ASIM's office for its first five years. The move to larger quarters on Geary Street (naturally, still in San Francisco) took place a few months after ASIM's fifth annual meeting. The Geary Street office telephone number—BA1-3131—was easy to dial in the days before push buttons. That office would be home to ASIM until 1968.

The 350 Post Street address located the headquarters office clearly enough. But the ASIM stationery of 1958 made it equally clear that much of the work of the young Society was carried out elsewhere: President Bullock, President-Elect Persons, and Executive Committee members Goss, Seigle, Wever and Yater, all had their names and personal office addresses printed at the top of the letterhead; only Secretary-Treasurer Callaway used the 350 Post address. Changing this practice over the next few years turned out to be a difficult problem for Clyde Greene and the expanding ASIM staff.

While a home base and competent staff are of paramount importance to a new organization, an even more critical need is for the financial means to support them and an expanding array of activities. Once again, ASIM's early leaders demonstrated a careful mix of prudence and adventure. The question of dues came up first at the Founders Meeting, and one of those present, DeWitt Burnham, addressed the issue:

"Dr. Bullock, I am proud to be a founding member of the new organization—and I will probably get my head cut off, but why don't we all contribute $10—those of us who are here as founders—and put it in and have some money to work with. . . . I'll put in mine." The suggestion was made a motion, was passed unanimously, and "Burnham made out the first check ever made to the ASIM." Incidentally, Claude Callaway, who had just had the title of Treasurer added to his previous election as Secretary, took the motion seriously: within ten days he sent follow-up letters (on CSIM stationery with California crossed out and American typed in) dunning those attendees who had failed to cough up the $10 at the meeting.

ASIM's first year, working as an Interim Committee until Bylaws could be approved at the first Annual Meeting in Boston in 1957, was supported by the Founder's contributions—and by the CSIM which had a $1,500 kitty it was willing to lend.

At the Boston meeting, it was "agreed that the dues of all Societies admitted, or tentatively admitted at this meeting, would be $3 for each member until July 1, 1957. After July 1, 1957, the regular dues of $10 per member would be payable." This recommendation was passed, but only after an amendment to make the amount $15 was beaten. Payment from some components was slow, but enough came in that by the time of an Executive Committee meeting in January 1958, Callaway reported that the Society was solvent. The early Bylaws said that the annual dues would be determined by the Council (later the Board of Trustees), but this important function was subsequently turned over to the House of Delegates. By the time of the second meeting in Atlantic City, George Wever, Finance Committee chairman, was able to report an anticipated balance of $18,360 for the end of the fiscal year.

This healthy state of affairs lasted for more than two years, but by the time of the 5th annual meeting in Miami Beach in May 1961, it was necessary to ask the House of Delegates to approve an increase in annual dues to $20 a member. The pace of activities had increased so rapidly that expenses had risen beyond expectations and Secretary-Treasurer Clyde Greene had to seek help from component societies by asking them to prepay dues for a short time in order to help the Society's cash flow.

The early leaders of ASIM clearly understood the importance of communications. In its first year, Mildred Coleman must have been pretty busy just keeping up with the spate of correspondence emanating from Bullock, Callaway, et al. And the many copies—to the Founding Group, to state SIM leaders, or just to involved internists out there—must have created no small mechanical problem in those days before inexpensive office copying machines.

Ordinary external communications—letters to other medical organizations, to health insurers, to government officials—were mostly a matter of dictating whenever the occasion seemed to demand it and mailing, along with copies to appropriate individuals or groups. But ASIM's early leaders were constantly alert to the need of communicating with another external group—the general public. Patients of internist members (and potential patients—not yet called "consumers") needed edification about the scope and limits of internal medicine. To this end, CSIM had earlier created a public relations committee, which had developed the "What Is an Internist?" leaflet and had promoted the famous Paul DeKruif *Readers' Digest* article.

One of the first committees appointed in the inchoate ASIM was for public relations. By late 1957, its chairman, Stewart Seigle, was able to display two finished products—the "Purposes of the American Society of Internal Medicine" and the "Guide for the State Society of Internal Medicine." The attendees at the 1958 annual meeting were so pleased with these products that they instructed the committee to distribute copies of both to top-echelon people at AMA and ACP.

Over the next several years, public relations continued to be a major effort of the national organization. The 1960 roster of committees shows that the Public Relations Committee had as many members (14) as the economics-oriented Medical Services Committee. In 1961, the Public Relations Committee Chairman, Malcolm S.M. Watts, wrote a column for the newsletter (possibly in response to criticisms from the outside that ASIM was chiefly concerned about dollars) in which he defended the Society's emphasis on economics, pointing out that, from the public's point of view, it should be attributed not to greed but to a concern for the quality of patient care.

Efforts to educate the public about internal medicine also surfaced in a number of the component societies, in which scholarly internists lent their literary talents to trying to improve the CSIM's original leaflet "What Is an Internist?" A memorable example took place in New York, where NYSSIM leaders John Williams and Herbert Berger combined to produce a glossy brochure entitled "Your Doctor Is an Internist." It was so good that ASIM (even with its heavy weight of Californians) saw fit to advertise the availability of the New York product to all ASIM members.

In 1960, a resolution from public relations-minded NYSSIM was passed, asking study of the feasibility of hiring expert public relations consultants to help ASIM disseminate its word. When nothing happened, a year later the NYSSIM delegation maneuvered to tie the dues increase in with an expanded PR program. When no visible progress ensued, NYSSIM gave up and decided to do its own thing—a decision that would result in a NYSSIM-sponsored movie production—in color—showing an internist (looking for all the world like John Williams) at work solving a patient's diagnostic problem.

If "external" communications were deemed important, so was the need recognized to keep members of the new organization informed about what was going on. Once a master list of the members of the charter component societies was developed (after the 1957 Boston meeting), and once addressograph plates were made, it was easy for ASIM officers to send their important news directly, instead of relying on component secretaries to get the word out. And the expense of such a mailing—3,500 members times a three cent stamp—was affordable even for a tightly budgeted society like ASIM. Bullock and Callaway each took advantage of this route. When Elbert Persons was elected president in 1958, one of his first actions was to write a four page

AMERICAN SOCIETY OF INTERNAL MEDICINE
ASIM
INCORPORATED APRIL 18, 1958
A CALIFORNIA NON-PROFIT
CORPORATION

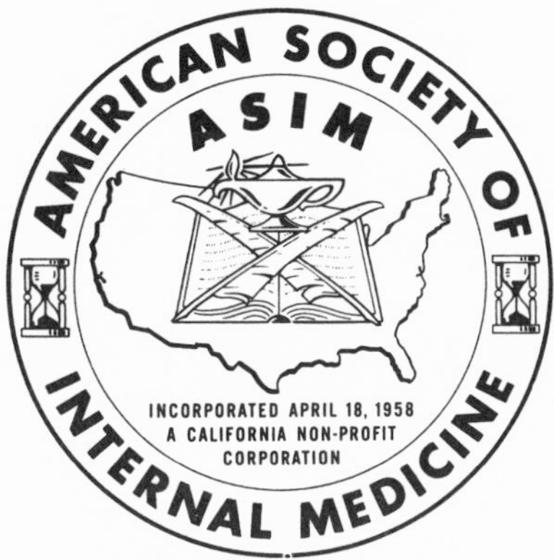

State-Of-The-Society message to all members. Subsequent presidents often continued this practice.

But more was needed, some regular route for informing members of what was going on. A prototype newsletter—even though it was sent only to component presidents and secretaries—was composed and distributed by Assistant Secretary-Treasurer Clyde Greene in October, 1958. Four pages long, it was full of news: the appointment of Richards as Executive Secretary, future annual meetings, growth (ASIM had reached 4907 members and 40 components—although only 23 of the latter had paid their dues), brochures (revisions of "Purposes" and "What Is an Internist?") and other items. One item had to do with a seal which Greene described in this poignant but fatalistic fashion: "The new seal of ASIM, shown on the first page, is a combination of geography and a daydream about the symbolic representation of an internist's chores. Thus we have the lamp of learning lighting the implements of study, writing and reflection. As a final stroke the hourglasses point out that a good work-up requires at least an hour of time. Seals are carefully scrutinized by those responsible for their adoption, then are affixed to thousands of documents and never carefully looked at again. So let it be with this one."

The newsletter also announced that wallet-sized membership cards had been printed and could be obtained by component societies (if they were willing to cough up $3.50 per hundred) for distribution to active members. The newsletter also reported that membership certificates—for components to distribute to their members—had been prepared, "handsomely printed in blue and gold." The certificates were to become something of a controversy—what if a member later dropped out, through malfeasance or failure to pay dues? Would the certificate of membership still hang in the malefactor's consulting room? A solution that was suggested was to make the certificate good only for a year, but the logistical problem of sending on an annual basis new dates for members in good standing to glue on their old certificates seemed insuperable. Thereafter, certificates stayed in force as a regular symbolic display of membership status, but as time went on they became less important.

By 1959 it seemed time to communicate with all the members of ASIM. Volume One, Number One of the ASIM *Newsletter* appeared in July of that year, containing announcements of meetings and activities. At first the *Newsletter* appeared six times a year, but in 1960 the Board decided to increase the frequency to ten times a year (the summer months in those days still being a time of diminished activity). The four-page *Newsletter* fulfilled its purpose: it was always chock-full of information about what was going on. There were pictures of people (officers, Trustees, speakers, staff) and places (a new headquarters office) and things (especially fee schedules). The text talked about ideas (editorials by presidents or executive directors) and people (who was serving on what committee, which Trustess had participated in what national meeting, who was invited to speak at the next annual meeting, and who were newly elected officers of which component). The cumulative effect on rank-and-file members must have been impressive. Readers could not escape the evidence that ASIM and its components comprised an organization that was both vigorous and effective in pleading the cause of internists and their patients.

8

Yearly Meetings
Annual Assemblages

By the time of ASIM's fifth birthday—the annual meeting of May, 1961, held in Miami Beach—this bustling bastion of internists had come a long way from the Founders Meeting. From a simple notion—a perceived need by a group of internists in one state—had come an organization that, by dint of rational discourse and hard work, had compiled a remarkable list of accomplishments, one sufficient to establish ASIM as a bright star in the firmament of health care.

One way to tot up accomplishments during those five years is to look back at ASIM's birthdays, the annual meetings that marked a point for pausing and assessing the Society's past, present and future.

The inchoate Society, living in limbo for a year, had functioned only as an Interim Committee—albeit under the vigorous direction of its chairman, Lewis Bullock—until a formal structure could be created. The first order of business in Boston in April 1957 was to discuss, amend, and ultimately approve a set of Bylaws that had been provisionally prepared by Goss, Gilbert and Seigle. The second item was to put flesh on the skeleton; Bert Persons presented the report of his Admissions Committee. California, North Carolina, Washington, Florida, New Mexico, Arizona, District of Columbia, Connecticut, Michigan, Idaho and Oregon had their applications in order and were accepted first (with a combined total of 1,997 individual members). Utah, Hawaii, New Jersey, Mississippi, New York and Minnesota (totaling 647 members) had just completed admission requirements and were accepted during the meeting. Alabama, Oklahoma, South Carolina and South Dakota were admitted pending completion of requirements. Nebraska, Kentucky, West Virginia, Maine, Wisconsin and Ohio, all coveting the distinction of counting their constituents as charter members, sought from the floor and won approval of that honor. By meeting's end, ASIM—more or less in technical compliance with the new Bylaws—was an official body, made up of 27 states and some 3,500 members.

The third item was to insure continuity of vigorous leadership. The newly appointed delegates approved the report of the nominating committee: for president, Lewis Bullock; for president-elect, Elbert Persons; for secretary-treasurer, Claude P. Callaway; for Executive Committee members, Clark Goss, Stewart Seigle, George Wever and Wallace Yater.

This baptismal meeting gave the Society form and substance.

During the next year, ASIM had added nine more component societies—Illinois, Indiana, Louisiana, Maryland, Massachusetts, Missouri, North Dakota, Tennessee, and Wyoming—and had grown to some 4,500 members. During the April 1958 meeting in Atlantic City, four more components—Montana, Puerto Rico, South Carolina, and Virginia—were added. Hawaii was kept as an active society when its then president, Elmer Johnson, paid the entire membership dues for the preceding year out of his own pocket.

Reports of committee activities were presented in detail. Legislative Committee Chairman Bill Walsh reviewed the "many items of legislation which may affect the practice of internal medicine." Clark Goss reported for his Medical Services Committee in relation to fee schedules. Bert Persons detailed the work of the Membership (formerly Admission) Committee. Fred Hnat proposed some Bylaws improvements. Stewart Seigle described the output of the Public Relations Committee. And George Wever recounted the positive state of the Society's finances and proposed a budget of $51,488.83 for the following fiscal year.

For the first time, program speakers were heard. Wallace Yater, simultaneously a Trustee of ASIM and secretary general of the ACP, spoke optimistically about "The Future of Internal Medicine and the Relationship of the ACP to the ASIM." William Alan Richardson, editor of *Medical Economics* magazine, dealt—at a pragmatic and less sanguine level—with "The Changing Status of The Internist in Health Insurance Practice."

Elbert Persons ascended to the presidency and the energetic and peripatetic Clark Goss was voted president-elect. George Wever, who had chaired the meeting of the Founding Committee two years earlier replaced Claude Callaway as secretary-treasurer, and Clyde Greene won his first ASIM office as assistant secretary-treasurer (he would continue in one capacity or another through his past presidency year in 1971).

By April 1959, ASIM was becoming a more sophisticated and complete organization. Only two additional components, Georgia and Texas, had been added, but total membership continued to rise to about 5,400 internists. An executive director had been hired and the Board of Trustees was expanded to six persons (Donegan, Lehnhoff, Longley, Pollard, Wever, and Yater), in addition to the four officers.

Clark Goss took over as president at the Chicago meeting, and Connecticut's Stewart Seigle, ASIM's articulate spokesman in Congressional testimony as well as a host of public relations and communications feats, became president-elect during Goss' tenure as president. Greene became secretary-treasurer, a position he would hold for many years.

The House debated eight resolutions dealing with structure (Bylaws amendments) and function (fee schedules, public relations, legislation, etc.) and managed to accomplish all of its business in one day: First session 9:00-10:45 a.m., Second session 3:45-5:00 p.m.

The program included prominent national figures, talking about health insurance and relative value schedules. But the feature was a panel, moderated by George Wever and including as panelists Lewis Bullock, Charles K. Donegan, James W. Hall, and Chester S. Keefer, discussing the intriguing topic of "What An Internist Must Do, What He May Do, and What He May Not Do."

The Meetings Committee thought highly enough of the program session for the April 1960 meeting in San Francisco to give it a somewhat sweeping thematic title: "The Scientific, Social, Economic and Political Responsibilities of the Internist." The Committee must have been of the opinion that panels were a better educational medium than solo speakers; it arranged no fewer than three such. One focused on "Public Relations of the Internist," including a lay expert, Walter Barlow, president of the Opinion Research Corporation of New Jersey (inadvertently broadcast by the Palace Hotel to every room in the building), an AMA spokesman, and two ASIM advocates of public relations, New York's redoubtable John Williams and Massachusetts' professorial Howard Root. A second panel dealt with liaison activities and included two outsiders and two ASIM experts, Claude Callaway (on state medical associations and specialty societies) and Pennsylvania's Wendell Gordon (on Blue Shield). The third panel, dealing with the practice aspects of internal medicine, featured Dwight Wilbur as keynote speaker, and Ross Taylor among other panelists.

Honored guests included Howard P. Lewis, ACP's president, and Edward Rosenow, its executive secretary. Featured luncheon speaker was William B. Walsh, former chairman of ASIM's legislative committee and now president of the Eisenhower-blessed Project Hope.

Five more components were added—Colorado and Iowa (in October 1959) and Arkansas, Delaware and Vermont at the meeting. A directory of members had been published for the first time in 1959, and shortly after this annual meeting a printed insert was distributed to all members. The six-page insert showed that Michigan's Ross V. Taylor had been voted president-elect (to serve with President Seigle, Immediate Past President Goss and Secretary-Treasurer Greene). The six

Trustees included incumbents Lehnoff, Longley, Donegan, and Wever, and two new ones, Massachusetts' Howard Root and New York's Robert Westlake. The 47 components were listed, along with their presidents and secretaries. Fourteen committees (ACP Liaison, Ad Hoc Study, Annual Meeting, Bylaws, Education and Research Foundation, Finance, History, Legislation, Liaison, Medical Services, Membership, National Industrial and Labor Relations, Nominating, and Public Relations) were listed, as were the 97 members who worked on them. Medical Services and Public Relations tied for the highest number—14 each—and presumably for the top of the Society's priority list.

In Miami Beach in May 1961, the House of Delegates had so much business to consider—reports from officers and committees and a new record of twelve resolutions—that it met in first session on Saturday morning at 10:30 and reconvened to finish its work at 2:00 p.m. on Sunday. In between, three reference committees met to consider reports and resolutions and to propose suggested outcomes. But the delegates (61 from 33 components) took their work seriously, refusing to give pro forma approval and insisting on amendments to modify language and, not infrequently, substance.

Among the subject matters discussed and resolved were: legislation (support of AMA's program for care for the aged, support of implementation of Kerr-Mills legislation, and opposition to the proposed King-Anderson bill); medical services (adoption of a resolution entitled "Descriptive Coding of Medical Services" and of a plan for submitting it to the June meeting of the AMA House); liaison (support of an effort to establish better relationships with the American College of Surgeons); public relations (recommendation that ASIM seek advice from professional public relations firms); internal affairs (approval of some housekeeping Bylaws changes, and adoption—without dissent—of a doubling of the dues rate to $20.00, of which $18.00 would be used for the general budget and $2.00 would be set aside for a special reserve fund. While all of these topics were standard grist for the five-year-old ASIM mill, there was one new direction that surfaced: Resolution #5, entitled "Enforcement of Medical Standards," asked ASIM to recommend to the ACP that they work together "in the establishment of a pilot study to audit the hospital and office medical records of members of ASIM." Twenty years later, the organizations would be midway through the implementation of the PIQuA (Private Initiative in Quality Assurance) project, designed to accomplish just that purpose.

Missouri's Maxwell Berry and Pennsylvania's Wendell Gordon were elected as new Trustees, and George Wever, part of the ASIM venture since the beginning, was honored by being chosen president-elect. Unfortunately, he shortly thereafter suffered a major myocardial infarction (when flying in an unpressurized plane to a component society meeting in Idaho); his internist advised him not to serve, his place was taken by Florida's young Charles Donegan, and Californian Malcolm Watts was added to the list of Trustees. When past presidents later decided to form a club within a club, they honored Wever by calling it the George Wever Club.

The Meetings Committee's fondness for sweeping themes showed up again; the title of the program session was simply "Internal Medicine and Society Today." Representatives from labor, organized medicine (AMA's President-Elect Leonard Larson), hospital administration (Walter J. McNerney, later to head national Blue Cross and Blue Shield) and government (the Special Assistant to the Secretary of HEW bore the euphonious name of Boisfeuillet Jones) all participated in a panel on the meeting's theme. Another panel, featuring Wever and Donegan, asked "Can We Improve Medical Care? Can We Reduce The Cost?" The two-year-old Federal Employees Health Benefits Act got a presentation from its director. Trustee Lehnhoff discussed "Relationships Between ASIM and Its Component Societies." ACP's president Chester Keefer,who had recently written a glowing article for the *New England Journal of Medicine* about the healthy relationships between ACP and ASIM, was the featured luncheon speaker.

One more component—Kansas—was added to the list, bringing the total to 48 and the number of members to 7,450.

Afterthought

By its fifth birthday, ASIM had come a long way indeed. In terms of size of membership, it was in the top six or seven among specialty societies. In regard to reputation, its leaders were acknowledged in the arenas of organized medicine, government and third-party payors to be resourceful, forceful, and sensible spokesmen for internal medicine. As far as accomplishments were concerned, it had built an effective organizational federation in a short period of time. Within a few months it would achieve a great victory, to get the AMA House of Delegates and later the National Association of Blue Shield Plans to recognize the need to be specific about medical (nonsurgical) services.

There was still a long way to go. The special nature of the services of internists was not yet widely recognized; and those services were not yet acknowledged in the practical sense of routine payment for them. ASIM leaders were still supplicants, knocking on doors to try to get their case heard. It would be some years before any other segment in the health care arena would automatically turn to ASIM for advice and consent; and it would be even longer until ASIM leaders would graduate into positions of higher responsibility throughout the health care enterprise.

Five years after its founding there were early signs of a modest shift in ASIM's strategy and posture. A new second wave of younger leaders was appearing, coming up through the ranks of component societies and national committees. They showed a tendency to adopt a less adversarial, some might call it more statesmanlike, approach to dealing with issues and people. And their focus of attention was shifting from a principal emphasis on economic matters to a new interest in the factors influencing the quality of medical care.

ASIM was evolving, slowly but surely, into a new mode.

VOLUME II

The Growing Years

Adolescence and Adaptation

Aphorism: Evolution

"EVOLUTION: A process of gradual and relatively peaceful social, political, and economic advance."

As usual, Webster has a way of capturing essentials. The years between ASIM's fifth and fifteenth annual meetings—roughly, the decade of the sixties—were a time of immense change for the young Society. The more visible yardstick of that change was simple growth, an arithmetical increase in the numbers of members, component societies, dollars in the budget, programs, meetings, and staff.

But with growth comes responsibility. ASIM had to learn to deal with its thousands of members and dozens of component societies, not only to take from them, in terms of human and fiscal resources, but also to return something to them in terms of tangible and intangible benefits. Much of ASIM's time and energy during the sixties was devoted to strengthening its relationships with its component societies and with its rank-and-file members.

ASIM grew during the sixties in another, more subtle way, in its unfolding capacity to respond effectively to environmental stresses and fluctuations. In short, ASIM's growth was an evolutionary one, and Webster's definition captures remarkably well the essence of the Society's approach during those years.

Certainly, the decade of the sixties was a time of profound social, political, and economic change in the health care arena. It was the era of the Great Society, when the resources necessary to effect social change seemed inexhaustible. The result was the swift passage of legislation to finance medical care for the aged and the poor, and the involvement of government in the planning, development, research, and evaluation of health services. It was a time of recognition of shortages of medical professionals and of resolve to take corrective action. It was a time of beginning discussions of professional accountability and of a search for ways to demonstrate to the public the profession's sense of responsibility for the quality of care. And, it was a time of intra-professional misunderstanding and sometimes squabbling.

To all of these stimuli, ASIM managed to respond. While it is likely that the ASIM leaders involved in the era would insist that it was marked by turbulence and crisis, the fact is (as seen through history's softer focus) that events really were "gradual and relatively peaceful." Certainly, ASIM's responses were never hasty nor ill-conceived. The internist's deliberate process of analysis and synthesis was applied to events and yielded a considered and rational position that could stand up against close scrutiny and opposition. ASIM became known, in the halls of Congress and in the circles of organized medicine, as an organization with thoughtful and well-presented positions.

Webster said it well. ASIM during the sixties showed remarkable evidence of "social, political, and economic advance."

1

The Membership
Agreeable Additions

The sine qua non of a successful professional organization is a sizable membership. It is helpful if significant numbers of members are willing to participate actively in organizational affairs, but the critical mass is made up of rank-and-file (also called "grassroots") members who neither desire to serve on committees nor aspire to leadership roles, but who are sufficiently convinced of the merits of the organization and of the benefits deriving to them that they are willing to pay dues on a recurring basis.

In both respects, ASIM did well in the sixties. Members willing to assume leadership roles were not hard to find in those halcyon days. The component societies—their number rose to 50 by the end of this decade—regularly came forth with people of talent, energy, and ambition, who were willing to enter the local fray at a top position or to serve simply as a member of a national committee. Not a few future ASIM leaders simply appeared on the scene, happening on a committee session at an annual meeting (attended perhaps because of a contiguous ACP session), expressing an opinion, and finding themselves suddenly a member of the committee. Still others were bright young internists sharing a practice with, or perhaps just living in the same town as, a senior ASIM leader; having shown signs of worth, they would shortly be pressed into service by their colleagues. Whatever the portal of entry, a sufficient number of leadership types floated to the top that ASIM nationally, and its component state societies, had access to a large cadre of workers willing to lend their considerable talents to advancing the cause of internists and their patients.

ASIM also did well in terms of attracting rank-and-file members, and membership rose to more than 10,000 by 1971. Some of this growth came from the word getting around about the new and energetic society that was taking up the cudgels for internists. Not infrequently, letters inquiring about how to become a member would simply show up "over the transom." More often, active recruitment measures were needed to bring new members into the fold. Different component societies tried different approaches, including direct mail appeals, but it was soon recognized that the best results were achieved with a one-to-one appeal: one already-converted internist proselytizing his partners, associates, fellow staff members, etc. Negative reactions were rarely encountered and potential members, once jawboned by a colleague, usually became dues-paying members. The difficult part, from a membership chairman's viewpoint, was to inspire current members sufficiently that they would take up the jawboning process.

The criteria for membership were generally straightforward: a candidate had to be a true internist practicing at a level of competence acknowledged by peers. To be sure there were endless debates about whether or not to require Board certification or Fellowship in the College, and there was some variation among the component societies as to how rigidly they held to these criteria, but in general what was wanted was a good practicing internist.

The mechanism for processing candidates was a little cumbersome, requiring a detailed form to be filled out, a nominating letter, a seconding letter, endorsement by local peers, then approval by the component's governing body. The process sometimes took so long that a willing applicant would not win membership for months—a delay which often irritated the applicant and always irked the income-hungry treasurer of the component society. Countless hours of committee work were expended, at both the national and local levels, to streamline the process and shorten the decision-making time.

Despite these difficulties, the membership rosters expanded steadily during the sixties. That major evidence of success—annual renewals—was healthy enough that membership graphs showed a nearly straight line upward slope.

Admittedly, with each increase in dues, the line shows a modest, temporary dip, but never to the degree anticipated by prophets of doom arguing to the Board or the House against the proposed increase. In 1967, when a dues increment of $20 was proposed by the Finance Committee, the Board, apprehensive that an economy-minded House might turn down the proposal, devised a tactic to convince the delegates of the essential nature of the broad scope of activity being carried on by the Society. Joseph Painter, then chairman of the Medical Services Council, was assigned to display for the House's edification every single activity taken by his Council and its member committees for the preceding year. This he did, in such exquisite and lulling detail that Joe's wife insists, perhaps apocryphally, that she listened to the first part of his report, went out to lunch with "the girls" and returned to find him still talking. The tactic worked; once the filibustering fog lifted, the narcotized House passed the dues motion without protest.

But despite ASIM's evident success in attracting and retaining members, there were still hungry membership chairmen who wanted more. During the sixties, several attempts were made to add a separate class of members to be called "associates." At one time this meant non-internist physicians, in emulation of the ACP's practice of taking in worthy pathologists, dermatologists, psychiatrists, radiologists, or neurologists (i.e., other "non-cutting" doctors). Such efforts were always defeated by the argument that ASIM's very name meant it had to be limited to internists. Not until 1977 would the House finally agree that neurologists, whose training parallels that of internists in many respects, could qualify for membership.

The "associate" category (in this case also called "candidate") was similarly advocated off and on for internists-to-be, those young physicians still in residency training who would later be almost certain to qualify for active membership. Get them on board, the argument went, and they would learn early about ASIM activities and subsequently stay on as regular members. The notion was finally accepted in 1966 to admit residents into non-dues-paying special membership that would require later conversion to active status. Ensuing membership campaigns met with modest success. The College's better record is perhaps partly attributable to its greater charisma to residents, but also at least in part to a free subscription to the *Annals of Internal Medicine*.

But there were still mature, active internists out there who had somehow not conceded the desirability of joining ASIM. Many of these were subspecialists and, not surprisingly, they tended to find more worth in their cardiology or gastroenterology or hematology organizations than in a society that seemed more involved with "general" internal medicine. For whatever reason, campaigns to attract individual subspecialists into ASIM membership were not very successful, and ASIM leaders decided that some benefits might accrue to ASIM from closer liaison with specialty societies. Tennessee's Ben Hall was assigned this task when he came on the Board in 1971 and he succeeded in developing a Subspecialty Council, made up of a number of subspecialty organizations, which met occasionally under ASIM's sponsorship to discuss matters of mutual concern. There was an initial burst of enthusiasm, but this soon waned and only the neurologists showed a continuing verve for ASIM's approach.

The greatest effort of all was expended in trying to attract one particular segment of the internal medicine population—the cohort of academic internists. These individuals (themselves often subspecialists) carried out their work in medical schools and associated hospitals, devoting themselves in varying proportions to teaching, research, administration and practice, the last usually in the consultation mode. Virtually all academic internists were Board-certified and, as a matter of course, were usually Fellows of ACP; a fraction of them had leadership roles in those organizations. Winning them to ASIM's banner was no easy matter; they tended to care more about bioscience than the science of economics and not a few of them looked down their noses at such crass commercial pursuits as getting proper reimbursement for internists' services.

During the sixties, ASIM employed two different strategies to overcome this negativism. James Feffer's approach was to take advantage of the fact that the Medicare/Medicaid entitlements, because they paid for services to beneficiaries who were customarily occupants of teaching hospital beds, forced academicians willy-nilly to pay attention to reimbursement mechanisms. Feffer's strategy was simple: ASIM should use its expertise to develop some model "practice plans" for teaching hospitals, in which the academic attending staff could join together in a sort of group practice arrangement to administer the complex mechanics of collecting and distributing monies from third-party payors. A task force was formed, the model practice plans were developed and then offered to medical school deans. There was some penetration of the market and the plans did work (at least until Washington changed the rules). But apparently only a few academic internists saw all this as evidence of ASIM's expertise and therefore desirability; a trickle of new members signed up.

The Charlie Smyth strategy was different. The Colorado rheumatologist, himself a respected academic, had early been persuaded of the righteousness and timeliness of ASIM's message, and he landed on the Board of Trustees in 1967. A warm and winning man, he employed the simplest of strategies to win over his academic colleagues: in his travels to meetings, he used the old one-to-one approach and, answering each wavering objection firmly, simply convinced his listener of the merits of ASIM. This personal approach had some success: there was a measurable increase in academic internists who signed up. But their retention was less than perfect, and when Smyth finished his tour on the Board, the strategy fell into disrepair.

This is not to say that there were not other academics who, like Charlie Smyth, perceived something worthwhile in ASIM. Peter Talso, then chairman of the department of medicine at Illinois Loyola's Stritch Medical School was a gargantuan advocate of socioeconomic expertise who ended up on the Board from 1964 until 1967, when illness forced him to curtail his activities. Other component societies tried with varying success to persuade local medical school professors to join up. ACP leaders, with a few notable exceptions, were ASIM members and, with varying degrees of persuasiveness, talked up its virtues to College members and Fellows. But the fact is that academia in general—that hierarchy of assistant, associate and full professors of medicine in medical schools—and the subspecialty-oriented attending staffs of medical departments of teaching hospitals were simply not attracted to ASIM's banner.

It is an interesting sidelight that ASIM made no special effort to court membership proposals for internists who happened to be female. The reason undoubtedly lay in the fact that there were not very many of them; exact statistics are not available, but it is likely that only three to four percent of internists in the sixties were women. But, while ASIM's members were predominantly of the male gender, a number of excellent women internists worked hard on its behalf. In California, Roberta Fenlon was a president of the California Medical Association and served on various ASIM committees in the sixties; in 1971 she was honored by being awarded the title of Distinguished Internist of the Year. Another California woman was Charlotte Baer who rose to prominence in the late sixties for her peer review activities. She served with distinction on ASIM's Peer Review Council; her brillant career came to an abrupt end with her untimely death in 1973. Katherine Borkovich of Baltimore, a member of ASIM since its inception and a founder of the Maryland Society of Internal Medicine, served in many positions for both societies. She, too, was honored as ASIM's Distinguished Internist, in 1978.

One final category had to be considered for membership in ASIM. These were individual practitioners who called themselves internists in the AMA's periodic survey of physicians but whose credentials were not impeccable. Many of these self-designated internists were general practitioners who had decided to give up (or who had been forced by specialists on their hospital medical staff to give up) their surgery and obstetrics; there being no slot for "general medicine" in the AMA list of practice categories, what could be more natural for such physicians (particularly those who might have had a year or two of medical residency training) than to give themselves a step up by claiming they practiced internal medicine. This practice caught some component society membership chairmen in the dilemma of simultaneously wanting to expand the roster of members and striving to keep standards up. Happily, component governing bodies opted for high standards. Some insisted on ABIM certification as the mark of excellence, but most settled for unequivocal evidence of thorough training in a recognized residency in internal medicine. Eventually, the ABIM set standards for qualification to take the Board exam and issued letters to prospective candidates certifying their eligibility. This made a component membership chairman's job easier; if a potential ASIM member had such a letter, his educational credentials were satisfied.

Still, there was considerable variation among components as to strictness of criteria for membership. The bylaws of many of them still mentioned Board certification or College Fellowship as a principal measure of acceptability. James Feffer, during his presidency in 1967-68, took these inconsistencies on as a problem needing solution. To him, the credibility and status of ASIM depended on its having its own criteria for membership (the most important of which were training in internal medicine and peer acceptance) and on its not settling for the criteria established by and for other organizations. His campaign to get components to change their bylaws accordingly met with considerable, if not universal, success. (It was not until 1981 that New Jersey SIM finally gave up its strict requirement for Board certification.)

A convincing argument can be made that efforts to make technical adjustments in bylaws and to mount enthusiastic campaigns to attract special kinds of new members had only a marginal effect on the overall makeup of ASIM's swelling membership. By the mid-sixties it was clear that the Society was made up principally, despite the sprinkling of teachers, researchers, and administrators, of one kind of physician. ASIM was of, by, and for the practicing internist. But not all qualified practicing internists were necessarily Board-certified. By 1973, the number of ASIM members who were certified was 66 percent of the total. Nor did all ASIM members necessarily seek entrance to the College; in 1973, about 55 percent had, but the number varied from component to component. In some, especially the smaller ones, the internists were a collective breed and virtually all of them were ABIM certified, ACP Fellows and ASIM members. Idaho's William Forney got all but two of that state's internists to join ASIM. In 1962 Trustee Max Berry reported that "of the 209 physicians belonging to the ACP, 198 are members of the Missouri SIM." In Oklahoma, Art Schmidt and others worked successfully to get that state's internists, including the medical schools' department members, to work together harmoniously. Wisconsin, prodded by founding member Bob Gilbert and a succession of other hard workers, established cordial and solid relationships among virtually all of its internists.

Other states, even some with prestigious medical schools, managed to achieve harmony within internal medicine ranks. In Maryland, Katie Borkovich and William Speed worked with College Governor Sam Asper (later ACP president and in 1981 its deputy executive vice president) to establish a common voice for internal medicine. In Massachusetts, Frank Foster, Robert Fahey, Peter Contompasis and others struggled valiantly to establish friendly relationships with Harvard, Boston University and Tufts internists. In Pennsylvania, Wendell Gordon, Robert Pressman, Jerome Chamovitz, Ray Grandon, James Collins, William Kelly and others worked hard at the Philadelphia and Pittsburgh poles of their state; the annual PSIM meeting with its featured "Breakfast with the Professors" did much to cement relationships with medical school internists.

But in some states, especially the larger ones, harmony could not be achieved. In New York and Illinois and, to a lesser degree, California, the town-gown conflict (with ASIM's practicing internists representing town and the ACP's academics representing gown) smoldered despite repeated efforts to put out the fire. In 1963, of 900 Board-certified internists in Manhattan, only 25 were ASIM members.

Despite these difficulties, ASIM components successfully attracted increasing numbers of physicians to the fold. By the time of ASIM's 15th birthday at the Annual Meeting of 1971, the roster of its members had swelled to more than 10,000. By and large, they came from the ranks of practicing internists. Inevitably they shared common experiences and perceptions, and this homogeneity of background and daily activity served the purpose of channeling and focusing their sense of purpose. Their representatives in ASIM's House argued endlessly and sometimes heatedly about tactical detail, but their commonalities far outweighed their differences. During the 1960s, ASIM policies and actions truly came to represent the consensus voice of practicing internists.

ASIM leaders were always on the lookout for something tangible that would give the grassroots member some return on his investment of dues. An early example was a form, devised by an ASIM committee and offered on tear-off pads at cost, that members could use to get reimbursement from insurance companies for information they sent in regarding a patient's eligibility for insurance. A similar device, for use by those internists who performed life insurance examinations for insurers, provided a mechanism for submitting appropriate charges for those services. In the late sixties, a modest campaign by ASIM helped clarify the conditions of, and payment for, the determination-of-disability examinations performed by many internists and paid for by the federal government. ASIM even entered the hospital domain where internists often were called on to provide their expert services to populations of patients; one example was an ASIM pamphlet outlining proper administrative and financial arrangements between hospitals and internists reading electrocardiograms.

Another route for providing tangible member benefits lay with insurance programs. In the early years, ASIM had arranged with ACP that ASIM members could automatically qualify for enrollment in the College's array of insurance programs. Throughout the sixties, it was common practice at ASIM national and component meetings to have an exhibit table set aside for College insurance administrators to sell their services. Although ASIM entered—somewhat gingerly at first—into negotiations with a separate group of insurers to provide policies to its members in 1962, it was not until 1970 that ASIM finally stopped the coattails arrangement with the College. The package of insurance offerings to ASIM members, developed over the years by an ASIM committee after careful study of benefit and premium structure, grew methodically to include at first investment and retirement programs, and later life insurance, health insurance, disability insurance, and the like.

Although not all ASIM members partake of these offerings, those who do have been pleased with their coverage. ASIM has been satisfied with the effect of the insurance package: it has kept some members in the fold, it has helped ASIM and SEREF budgets modestly through a dividend routing option, and it has resulted in a nice spin-off benefit, the annual reception provided by the Jones and Babson administrators at ASIM annual meetings.

ASIM sought to help its members in other, more practice-oriented ways. From the beginning, committees were charged with devising ways and means of helping internists conduct their practices in more efficient and more effective ways. In the mid-sixties, when ASIM's operating structure was consolidated into Councils, one of the four was called Medical Practice. The reorganization of Council roles in the late sixties shifted many functions into new alignments, but the Council on Professional Practice was kept intact. One of its major thrusts, of course, was in the arena of coding and nomenclature. While ASIM leaders were conducting a national campaign to get the services of internists recognized by third parties, they never forgot that recognition would be meaningless unless individual practicing physicians made use of standard nomenclature in their daily work. An educational process to promote the use of Current Procedural Terminology (CPT) was clearly needed, and, to this end, an unceasing campaign—survey questionnaires, pamphlets, booklets, audiovisual displays—was mounted during the sixties to help individual internists understand how and when to use "prolonged detention," "extended office visit," "limited consultation," and other phrases that signified not just semantic niceties but real world patient care. Using California's pioneer Relative Value Schedule as the foundation and the AMA's CPT as the model, ASIM committees proceeded to develop the Society's own PTI (Procedural Terminology for Internists) and then mounted a thorough marketing campaign to get member internists to understand and use it.

But the internist's practice was much more than coding and nomenclature and getting reimbursed by third parties. A good internist also keeps good records. Countless committee hours were spent in efforts to help make that job easier and better. Early practice management committees concentrated on the development of forms, especially for recording the data from history-taking and physical examination, to facilitate good recordkeeping. The concept was easy to embrace, but its practical implementation was difficult. Advocates of the "clean sheet" approach argued with those who wanted to put everything on a printed form. Would check lists lead to cookbook medicine or would they remind the careful internist not to overlook anything? Astonishingly, consensus somehow was reached and several versions of the internist's history and physical form were put together, published, and offered for sale.

2

The Component Societies

Accretion of Affiliates

Development of strong component societies was a major thrust of ASIM during the sixties. Its structure as a federation, obviously based on the national model of the American Medical Association which similarly has both a national persona and a policy-setting group of delegates from constituent organizational subdivisions, was unusual among specialty societies. And ASIM was unique in placing such exceptional weight on the activities of its components.

During its first five years, most of ASIM's attention had been focused on the elementary process of signing up existing state societies of internal medicine and assisting at the birth of others in locales where no predecessor organization existed. By the early sixties, this process had largely been completed, although there would be stragglers added up until 1966 when Nevada and New Hampshire came into the fold.

Thereafter, the emphasis slowly changed. The ASIM leadership began to recognize that it did not suffice simply to put component societies in place and then leave them to their own devices. Some of them might have sufficient built-in energy to be self-starting and a few might even have enough resources—in terms of people and money—to conduct effective programs on their own. But most components were not so resourceful. Too many of them operated in fits and starts, alternating frenetic activity with long stretches of coasting inaction. It seemed component societies were, by and large, delicate plants, needing constant attention and nourishment if they were to be kept from withering and dying.

The ASIM Board and the members of ASIM's House of Delegates representing the component societies came to recognize that those components would need help if they were to become effective spokes in the ASIM wheel. Support would be needed in terms of expert advice and specific aid—and it would have to come from the national body.

The Board, it should be emphasized, never hesitated in mounting a support program. Not one Trustee offered the suggestion that the components were unimportant and that ASIM might be better off as a top-down organization like almost all other specialty societies. Indeed, ASIM leaders seemed truly to believe the theme that was heard in their speeches: The strength of ASIM lies in the strength of its component societies.

There were convincing points to be made in support of the rhetoric. Many of the socioeconomic and political problems that concerned internists took place not at the national level, but in the states, where governments were getting increasingly involved in health and where third-party payors operated with statewide rules. Working solely as a national organization, ASIM would be hard pressed to deal effectively with 50 different sets of circumstances. The local internist, on the other hand, would know the local players well (indeed, might even serve as their personal physician) and should be able to play the local game better—providing, of course, the know-how existed to play it at all.

But the component structure offered something even more important than the facility to carry out tasks on the local level. It provided the matrix through which the "bottom-up" structure of ASIM power was validated. Rank-and-file internists had direct access to their local leaders, both informally as colleagues and formally through the component's own policy-setting delegate system. In turn the component societies, in the give-and-take of ASIM's House of Delegates, actually decided the scope and limits of the policies of the national society. ASIM's officers and Trustees, while they enjoyed considerable freedom in making decisions between meetings of the House (nearly as much freedom as their opposite numbers in "top-down" specialty societies), were constrained to operate within the framework of existing policy and were constantly aware that if they strayed too far they would surely have to give an accounting before the House at its next meeting.

Some attempts to assist components had begun during ASIM's early years. An initial effort of Stewart Seigle's Public Relations Committee was to prepare two booklets. The first, of course, was entitled "The Aims and Purposes of ASIM," but, significantly, the second was called "Guide for State Societies of Internal Medicine." In the late fifties, sites for Board meetings were selected for geographical variation as well as to help fan some flames of enthusiasm among component societies in the region.

In 1961, ASIM launched the *Component Society Officers Bulletin (CSOB)*. The newsletter's purpose was obvious from its name: to inform component society leaders about what was going on, either events at the national level promising impact on the local or strategies working in one component that might have application in others. The *CSOB* was an immediate success and continues today to be an important channel of communication between ASIM and its components.

Another avenue developed more gradually. Individual ASIM Trustees naturally would retain a special interest in the progress of their states of origin and even occasionally in the affairs of neighboring states. Also, ASIM officers, in the natural course of things, would be invited to speak at a component society's annual meeting and, while there, would surely inquire about progress (or its lack), as well as offer advice about solving problems. These informal contacts were perceived by component leaders as remarkably helpful.

At the March 1963 meeting of the Board, an item called "Component Society Assistance" appeared on the agenda. The Trustees, recognizing the helpfulness of these informal contacts, discussed ways and means of applying them more widely and systematically. The solution was obvious: each Trustee would be assigned major responsibility for a number of component societies, at least to be available to them for consultation and, where indicated, to prod and stimulate them into action. The Trustee assignment plan was at first an informal one, but as time went on it became a highly structured, even rigid affair. Guidelines were drawn up for what Trustees were supposed to do for their assigned components, whom to call and when, what topics they were to inquire about, and what projects they should propose. They were expected to attend—and contribute to—the annual meeting of each assigned component, to deliver a speech at it (if invited) and, especially, to participate in the accompanying meeting of the component governing board. Since 1963, time has been set aside at every ASIM Board meeting to get reports (written, or at least oral) from each Trustee shepherd about his flocks.

The process of assigning each Trustee to a cadre of components is one of the chores of an incoming president, who is expected to take into consideration such items as geography and expense, as well as certain imponderables. For some reason, individual Trustees have always seemed to favor assignments to Puerto Rico and Hawaii over North Dakota and West Virginia. Another problem lies with how long to continue an assignment, since a single individual can serve on the Board as Trustee and officer for as long as nine years. Naturally, some doubt could arise about his ability to sustain continued effectiveness as an advisor over that long a period of time, particularly if it is the same component in which he happens to have spent a number of previous years as a state leader. It follows that some reshuffling of assignments should be beneficial, both to prevent boredom and possibly to allay antipathy on the part of component leaders.

One of the minor problems of the Trustee assignment policy relates to who pays for what. Under ASIM policy, ASIM picks up the expenses of officers traveling to components as invited speakers and of Trustees visiting their components on assignment. If a component chooses to ask another ASIM leader to be a featured speaker, it must pay for that privilege. The rule sounds simple, but questions of substitutions, cancellations, and alternate speakers have sometimes created situations requiring the wisdom of Solomon to adjudicate.

The strategy of traveling to the components has clearly been a workable and beneficial one. But so has the opposite approach of getting component representatives together at a special ASIM meeting designed for that purpose. In the early sixties, ASIM began to set aside time at national and regional meetings for component society workshops. A name closely associated with that period is Richard Bates, a Michigan internist whose style—suave, articulate, humorous—successfully kept the attention of component representatives as he led them through a participatory, give-and-take discussion of component problems and their solutions. Another successful scheme, based on the obvious observation that states like New York and California have different problems than, say, Wyoming and Arkansas, was to cluster leaders from similar-sized components together at a table to discuss their strategies with each other under the watchful guidance of one or more Trustees.

How did the components respond to all this effort? As might be expected, the effect—if it could somehow be measured in a hypothetical component activities index—varied all over the lot. In general, the small components needed the most help and prodding and the big ones the least, probably because size is directly correlated to the number of members in the talent pool, to say nothing of the material resources provided by dues revenues. Most components were neither large nor small, and consequently had middle-sized pools of talent and resources. To a considerable degree, their level of activities depended on the enthusiasm and energy of one or two individuals who characteristically would surface early and stay long in leadership posts.

Naturally, component societies that faced discrete problems tended to flourish, as their leaders gave evidence of willingness to grapple with—and often solve—difficult situations confronting internists. But if local problems were especially unique (and if problem-solving expertise to address them didn't exist within ASIM's national leadership), a component's feeling of identity with ASIM's mission would tend to flag. This may explain why Puerto Rico's involvement has not been a major one and why Canadian provincial societies of internal medicine (two of which had been represented at the Founders Meeting) never took hold as ASIM components. However, this reasoning does not explain why a few states—Vermont and Wyoming come to mind—have never achieved more than a token involvement with ASIM. The answer there probably rests with an eternal enemy of ASIM ardor: complacency among practicing internists, an overriding satisfaction with the status quo, and a compelling reluctance to get involved in anything other than patient care.

But by and large, internist leaders in component societies have cared and have been willing—even eager—to do battle with problems facing internists and their patients. Many have preferred to devote most of their energies to the homefront, to dealing with state Blue Shield or public health departments or social services departments. But many enjoyed participating in the national scene: at the 1969 meeting of the House, 88 delegates from 42 components were present.

3

The Leadership
Astonishing Abundance

If ASIM's internal growth during the sixties was manifested principally in the number of its members and in the strength of its state component societies, its external image—the face it turned to the health care world—was shown most clearly in its activities as a national organization and in the personalities and actions of its national leaders.

Observers of the political process agree that leaders have a way of rising up through the ranks, reaching positions of high responsibility, ultimately leaving their mark on the scene, their particular mix of personality traits, attitudes and behavior patterns—all at a particular point in history. In the most successful organizations, the right leader comes to the fore at the right time, bringing just the appropriate mix of leadership qualities to cope effectively with current events.

Such serendipitous surfacing of suitable leaders had happened to ASIM from its birth—and continued to take place during its growing years. Its fifth president, invested at the fifth Annual Meeting in 1961, was Michigan's Ross Taylor. Cool and unflappable, it was he who came up with a phrase to capture the essence of the ASIM message: "The quality and cost of medical care are inseparable."

The president-elect under Taylor, George Wever, a Stockton, California internist and chairman of the 1956 Founders Meeting, was kept from his succession by a major heart attack. To replace him, ASIM found a young Florida internist who had been sitting on the Board since 1959. Soft-spoken but resolute, Charles Donegan brought youth (at age 42, he was then, and still is, the youngest ever to achieve ASIM's highest position) and boundless energy to the Society's expansion.

In 1963, it was Kansas City's Maxwell Berry whose mid-western common sense helped ASIM put out a bonfire in its relationship with the College and who helped add "social" to the Society's "economic" concern.

In 1964, a year of marked change in the nation's political and social climate, the Society went back to its San Francisco roots and elected Malcolm S. M. Watts as president. His special brand of intellectual and problem-solving skills were just right, both to channel the ongoing socioeconomic currents of ASIM activity and, especially, to guide the Society into a new course within the national legislative arena.

Nineteen sixty-five was the year of Medicare and Medicaid legislation and ASIM, needing administrative know-how to guide its response to the perceived impact of the new laws on internists and their patients, found it in New York's Robert Westlake, who brought finely honed management skills to the task of making the Society more efficient and effective.

A somewhat quieter year followed, one calling for consolidating and stabilizing traits. Personifying the necessary attributes of relaxed warmth was Pennsylvania's Wendell Gordon, who bent his efforts particularly to strengthening ASIM's ties with the rest of organized medicine.

Turbulence returned in 1967, in the form of a crisis in understanding between ASIM and ACP, along with a host of other loose ends needing tying up. Energy, strength of purpose, and decisiveness of action were needed, and Washington, D.C.'s James Feffer supplied those qualities in abundance.

Nebraska's Robert Long, ASIM's president in 1968, brought combined skills to the position, reemphasizing the Society's traditional focus on health insurance, fee schedules and procedural terminology, while simultaneously fostering its new interest in such things as computerized records and peer review.

In 1969, San Francisco's Clyde Greene was honored for his long years of service to the Society by being elected its thirteenth president. Articulate (and devoted to talking over the telephone), he led ASIM to pursue an eclectic variety of interests, ranging from improving internal structure and function to fostering external relationships with government and with other elements in organized medicine.

Presiding over the Society during the year leading up to its fifteenth birthday in March 1971 was Houston's Joseph Painter. Hard-working and devoted to detail, he was at the same time capable of conceptualizing in such arenas as peer review and what he called "the science of the delivery of medical care."

Unfortunately, not all of ASIM's leaders could become the Society's top officer. A host of other remarkable men served on its governing body, each bringing his own particular mix of qualities to the enterprise, simultaneously shoring up the strengths and buttressing the weaknesses of the top dogs. In the fifties, Henry Lehnhoff of Nebraska, H. Marvin Pollard of Michigan, Philip Longley of Ohio and Howard Root of Boston had all served in this capacity with distinction.

During the sixties a prominent figure was Wisconsin's Robert Gilbert. Attendee at the Founders Meeting, he was on the Board from 1962 to 1968, serving for much of that time as the Society's promoter of membership growth and watchdog over its fiscal books. Another luminary was Frank Foster (who in 1972 would be named ASIM Distinguished Internist of the Year) from Boston's Lahey Clinic, adding some strong AMA ties and some New England rectitude to Society activities. Carter Smith, courtly gentleman of Atlanta, in 1961 had submitted ASIM's resolution on non-surgical services to the AMA House, and served on the ASIM Board in the mid-sixties. Illinois' Peter Talso and Denver's Charlie Smyth were both academicians who saw the worth of ASIM's objectives and contributed their special viewpoints to the Board during the sixties. New York's Charles Weller served on the Board from 1964 through 1968 and was its principal champion of, and expert on, the impact of modern technology on the delivery of medical care. California's Richard Wilbur (later deputy executive vice president of the AMA, assistant secretary for health of the Department of Defense, and now the EVP of the Council of Medical Specialty Societies) served with distinction from 1966-69; always at the cutting edge of things, he introduced and somehow got passed by the Board a resolution that there should be no smoking during Board meetings, thereby affecting considerably their atmosphere. Illinois' Charles Downing and North Carolina's Horace (Junie) Hodges both made notable contributions to the Board's deliberations during the sixties. And especially noteworthy was Blaine Hibbard who served on the Board from 1967 to 1973, the last three years as secretary-treasurer and member of the Executive Committee.

It should not be thought that ASIM's work at the national level was carried out exclusively by a small cadre of Trustees. Much of the programmatic activities—discussing issues, analyzing possible courses of action, defining strategies and identifying possible new policies—was conducted by committees. Right from the beginning there had been a number of standing committees: Medical Services, Legislation, Public Relations, Membership, Finance, etc. Often, the pump was primed on these committees by a key individual, not infrequently a Trustee, who left an indelible mark of his effort. Medical Services, for example, owed its successes to the energies and expertise of James Feffer for the early part of the decade and of Joseph Painter for the latter. Similarly, Public Relations, which had been Stewart Seigle's bailiwick in the fifties, became Malcolm Watts' special province in the early sixties. ASIM's legislative concerns, shepherded by non-Trustee William Walsh in the early years, fell under Malcolm Watts' aegis as the Great Society legislation appeared, and later shifted to the individual who would be ASIM's "man in Washington" for nearly ten years—William Felts. Membership and Finance both bore the stamp of Wisconsin's Robert Gilbert for a good share of the decade of the sixties.

Although these committees' accomplishments carried the personality imprint of these strong leaders, the truth is that much of the committees' work was carried out by subcommittees, many of which had equally strong chairmen, individuals who never became Trustees but who nonetheless left their distinctive marks on ASIM's work. It was Ohio's Leonard Caccamo who supplied the creative effort behind the *Socio-Economic Handbook*. New York's John Williams personally sparked the creation of ASIM's movie "Case History," along with a host of other public relations and communications efforts. ASIM practice management aids for member internists were developed over the course of years by such dedicated individuals as Missouri's Frank Maple, Oregon's Estill Dietz and Wisconsin's late Addis Costello. (The latter had two other claims to fame. First, he kept track of the number of times he dealt with patient problems on the telephone, the result being the astonishing total of 4,300 times a year. Second, he enlivened many Wisconsin SIM meetings and an occasional ASIM meeting with ear splitting nocturnal playings of his beloved bagpipes.) ASIM also surfaced computer experts other than Charles Weller, including Philadelphia's Sidney Krasnoff, Kentucky's Irving Kanner and Hawaii's Fred Gilbert. Useful contacts with organized labor were made by Missouri's Frank Maple and John Berry, and ASIM's insurance and retirement programs for its members carry the unmistakable signature of Oregon's Harmon Harvey who chaired that committee for no less than 10 years.

As ASIM's scope of interests expanded, the number of appointed committees, subcommittees, ad hoc committees and task forces proliferated to the point of unwieldiness. In the early sixties, the Board, acknowledging the disarray and deciding that consolidation and grouping were indicated, reorganized itself into a Council structure. Four Councils, each with a cluster of committees, were organized, their broad arenas of responsibility being: Medical Practice, Medical Economics, Public Relations and Internal Affairs. In the late sixties, Otto Page chaired a Structure and Function Committee, which proposed a realignment. The new arrangement still had four Councils, and two of them—Internal Affairs and Professional Practice—were nearly identical with their predecessors in their committee substructure. But the other two Councils, perhaps reflecting a changing environment, were now called Liaison and Research/Development.

The Council structure undoubtedly added a degree of coordination and efficiency in budgeting and reporting mechanisms. But inevitably there were some overlaps, as well as some difficulty in fitting particular functions within the rigid structure. Government and legislation—arenas of growing importance to ASIM, especially from the mid-sixties on—always had trouble finding a suitable slot in any of the Councils; perhaps legislative concerns cut across all other arenas in haphazard fashion and are better left to ad hoc status.

During the sixties, John Gardner and other authors wrote about "organizational dry rot," the tendency for established organizations to lose their vitality and effectiveness, whether through leadership apathy or lack of foresight. ASIM's continuing youthful vigor and freedom from internal decay were never in doubt: During the 1960's, it paused no less than three times to reflect on where the Society had been and where it should be going.

The first planning session, in 1962, was informal, a meeting of the Board at which time was set aside from the hurly-burly of routine matters to review Society objectives and plans for achieving them.

The second was much more structured. In late 1966, a Long Range Planning Committee was appointed, made up of Malcolm Watts chairman, and members Clyde Greene, Blaine Hibbard, Wallace McCune of Pennsylvania, Joseph Painter, Beverly Paine of Michigan, Robert Raborn of Florida and Richard Wilbur. Its report, dated April 7, 1967, and addressed to the Board and to the House of Delegates (which later endorsed it), took 13 pages. It had a frontispiece, laying out in two paragraphs the place of internists and ASIM in the firmament:

> "ASIM is an organization of internists. The internist is a scholar with a practical bent. He is a scientist who is interested in people. He has a passion for thoroughness and for excellence and quality. He thinks in terms of diagnosis, treatment, prevention and rehabilitation. When he addresses these talents to the social, economic or political problems of delivering the best medical care to patients, he quickly achieves first respect and then leadership both in and out of the profession. This respect and recognized leadership are a predictable, even inescapable, result of these natural characteristics of the internist.
>
> "ASIM is the internist's organizational instrument through which he addresses himself to the public expectations for high quality health care and to the means by which these great expectations may be satisfied. ASIM is also an organizational instrument which must satisfy the expectations of its internist-members and provide them with a means to maintain and improve the excellence of their services and the efficiency with which they are rendered."

What followed was a series of 26 topics, each with a paragraph or two of discussion of the issues involved, after which came a specific recommendation outlining what ASIM should do about the subject. The list of topics was formidable: the public expectation and the private sector, central government and health care, a one-to-one patient-physician relationship, the new physician, identifying and describing internists' services, hospital privileges in internal medicine, hospital-centered health care, ASIM 'voluntary guidelines,' drug promotion, ASIM fact bulletin, office records and various forms, voluntary accreditation of internists, utilization of paramedical personnel, youth in ASIM, internists in training, the hospital-based internist, internists not in practice, involving the membership, communication through personal contact, a component society activities committee, regional activities for ASIM, annual meeting, ongoing long-range planning, planning for adequate financing, relationships with the American College of Physicians, and ASIM Foundation.

Not all recommendations received endorsement or subsequent implementation by the Board of Trustees; a few got token approval only and a couple were turned down flat. But most were received with enthusiasm and their recommendations were more or less promptly incorporated into action plans for the Society to undertake.

In May 1970, only three years later, a new ASIM Planning Report was published. This one was the work, not of a committee, but of the Board itself, which met for three days to hammer out its myriad details. The report bore the unmistakable mark of its principal author, President-Elect Joseph Painter. It was he who conceived the complex format for the discussions. It was he who drove the Trustees to cover all the issues in infinite detail, to the point where they had little time to enjoy the warm Bahama sun. (Sensitive to the possibility of being criticized for meeting in a luxurious resort outside the country, the individual Trustees paid out-of-pocket the $27.00 excess in travel expenses above what they would have paid had they stayed within continental boundaries.) And it was he who subsequently expounded on the report with its 40 pages of specifics.

The first 16-page section of the report identifies—in alphabetical order—a series of issues of importance to ASIM: cost, continuing education (both "socioeconomic" and "scientific"), delivery systems, efficiency, financing, manpower, quality, quantity, and technology. For each issue, a number of goals was delineated, and for each of these the necessary steps to achieve them and the locus within ASIM for carrying them through was spelled out. At the end of each issue, the proposed program items were recapitulated and value judgments made as to their priority level, urgency, deadline for achievement, estimated costs in terms of manpower and meeting time, need to work with other organizations, and the "solvability" likelihood.

To make sure no one missed the point, the remaining 24 pages of the report reshuffled all the material presented in the first section, this time organizing it by ASIM's internal structure and spelling out to each Council and committee its charge and a list of primary and secondary assignments, each with deadline and priority level assigned.

This planning report became the bible of ASIM committee work for several years thereafter (at least up until the time of the 1973 Planning Session). It behooved a conscientious committee chairman to open each meeting of his group with a review of progress or lack thereof with each item that had been assigned to its purview. ASIM staff, it is said, kept a huge chart occupying the better part of one wall displaying all the interlocking assignments within the ASIM hierarchy.

Another common problem of professional organizations is leadership turnover, in this instance meaning the exceedingly rapid processing of leaders through the system: a few years as Trustee, a year each as President-Elect, President and Past President—then disappearance from the scene. This rapid turnover has two ill effects. On the one hand, leaders can rise to exalted positions so quickly that they lack real-world seasoning. On the other, leaders of demonstrated competence can race through the process and in a few short years disappear from the stage, their wisdom lost. The syndrome includes several subsets, including the Past President's Ennui—the depression-inducing, traumatic 12-month trip from supreme power to oblivion. Then there is the President's Frenzy—the hectic, day-to-day pressure of activity that makes the trees so obtrusive that the forest loses its sharp focus. An especially prevalent subset, the President-Elect's Anxiety, occurs when young leaders skyrocket to high position—usually because of exceptional performance in a single locale or with a single issue—before they have had time to become familiar with the big picture or acquainted with other national leaders.

ASIM, employing as always the unique analytic skills of the internist, sensed the dangers of leader burnout and took appropriate preventive and therapeutic steps. One answer, authorized in 1969 and first implemented in 1970, was to appoint each year an Advisory Council whose members would be charged with giving the current Society leadership—at a one-or-two day retreat in a locale removed from everyday cares—some different perspectives about the health care enterprise, its issues, and its actors. For the first two years of its existence, the Advisory Council was made up exclusively of internists—young and old, practicing and academic—and they met with ASIM's current president, in this case Clyde Greene and then Joseph Painter (although the meeting was chaired by Past Presidents Feffer and Long.) In 1972, it was decided to broaden the base of Council membership to include non-internist perspectives, and to shift the spotlight from president to an earlier rung on the ASIM ladder—the president-elect. In the years since, the President-Elect's Advisory Council meeting—largely unstructured and with only the broadest of agendas—has included a host of notables from the health care arena, from the private and public sectors, insurers and consumers, ACP presidents and AMA presidents, young sprouts and old pros, congressmen and executive branch spokesmen, technologists and practitioners, theorists and pragmatists, economists and quality assessors. The outcome of this input from such an array of sources has been precisely what the ASIM prognosticators had anticipated. Little or no record has been kept of the words spoken at the PEAC conclaves, but it is clear that an unbroken string of Society presidents-elect have left their PEAC retreats with fresh perspectives and insights—and better prepared to take up the burdens ahead.

The threat of losing valuable input from competent leaders, shooting like a Roman candle through the ASIM hierarchy and seemingly destined for oblivion, was also dealt with by ASIM with characteristic orderliness. Perhaps cognizant of the opposite peril—leaders hanging on too long, staying in positions of power after their usefulness has passed, ASIM searched for and found a middle-of-the-road solution. In 1965, the George Wever Club was formed. It was named to honor the man who was chairman of the 1956 Founders Meeting and who, before a major heart attack, would have been the Society's sixth president. Its membership is both exclusive and elite. Every one has served as President of ASIM and is entitled to wear in his lapel the small gold gavel that is a symbol of former authority and responsibility. Theoretically, Club members can not only stay abreast of what is going on (they receive copies of important House and Board actions), they can also give voice to their views about those actions. Time is set aside at each Annual Meeting for the Club to convene so that its members can, should they see fit, take formal positions. Also, each member can attend meetings of the House and has the privilege of the floor. Practically, the Club's members seem loath to mix in with current events (the proposals to amalgamate with ACP in 1972 and to move to Washington in 1978 were notable exceptions to this generalization); in general, they prefer to enjoy the conviviality of joining with others of their select coterie, to reminisce, to grouse ("back in my day. . ."), and to make sentimental telephone calls to absent members.

ASIM had one more policy designed to make its decision-making capacity an effective one, scrupulously reflecting the consensus best efforts—even if transient—of the internist leadership. In a sense, this was a negative policy, designed to ensure that no single individual could hold, simply by virtue of tenure in a position over a long period of time, an ongoing latch on the balance of power. One way to accomplish this was to require that the executive director not come from the ranks of member internists. The thought was that, despite some possible advantages in background and perceptions that an internist might bring to the top staff job, the risk was greater that such a person might end up—whether meaning to or not—taking over more and more power from his transient and less sophisticated colleagues on the Board. Thus, although Clyde Greene's name, standing as it did for unassuming yet continually diligent service to ASIM, was twice mentioned as a possible paid staff executive, the decision was taken each time to search for a non-MD exec.

Perhaps an even more important method for guaranteeing the internist locus of decision-making was an unwritten but scrupulously observed policy about process, one that requires that all decisions must ultimately be made by vote of the full Board. In one context, this policy was designed to make sure that the Executive Committee of the Board could not take over the power of decision-making and leave the other Trustees as rubber-stamping figureheads; interim Executive Committee decisions must be ratified (and are sometimes reversed) by action of the entire Board. In another context, the policy serves to emphasize that the function of staff in the process of decision-making is to present information, to lay out options, even at times to proffer recommendations, but never to influence the decision. Bill Ramsey, ASIM's redoubtable executive since 1968, has placed great emphasis on this demarcation (even subsequent to 1978 when he was honored by having his title changed from executive director to executive vice president) and has insisted that his staff members observe it faithfully. This scrupulous separation of powers has served the purpose of placing the burden and responsibility of decision-making for ASIM directly on the shoulders of the Trustees. The policy must at times have been painful or frustrating for sophisticated, expert, full-time staffers watching a new Board member vote to re-invent the wheel. But wise old hands on the Board tend to prevail and the brash newcomer Trustee (undoubtably educated by staff in many small ways over time) in turn becomes a sophisticate. The policy seems to work.

4

The Quality Focus
Attesting Ability

Outsiders, inspecting this curious new Society with its exclusive interest in the socioeconomic aspects of health care, could probably be forgiven for expressing doubt if that interest was as devoted to "socio" as to "economic" matters. The casual observer, for instance, would have been correct in noting that ASIM's most visible early efforts were those directed at getting more equitable reimbursement to patients for their internists' services. But somebody observing the observers might also detect undertones of defensiveness, even envy, among certain of those critics who professed to see the Society as an upstart dealing only from crass commercial motives.

ASIM's original charter, the Constitution and Bylaws developed during its first year of existence, make frequent reference to the "quality" aspirations of the Society. ASIM's early pamphlet—"Aims and Purposes"—spelled out in no uncertain terms the Society's dedication to upholding the quality of care.

Furthermore, ASIM was not very old when its leaders spun off the Foundation for Socio-Economic Research and Education, which was charged, as its name suggests, with supporting projects that would place the delivery of medical care on a sound scientific basis. (For some reason, the Foundation was called just that in its early years; it was only in the sixties that switching the words around produced that euphonious acronym, SEREF, which, perhaps because of its faintly mysterious overtones of ancient mideastern wisdom, became the common appellation.)

One of the Foundation's early charges was to discuss with the University of Michigan a project to define the services of internal medicine in a way that would be precise enough to develop a valid relative value scale. By 1962, the ASIM Board allocated $5,100—no small sum in those non-affluent days—to the SEREF Board, which in turn awarded $5,000 (presumably keeping the extra $100 to keep its internal workings afloat) to the University of Michigan. After some delay, the University came up with a study proposal that was acceptable to the ASIM and SEREF Boards (at that time, the same people sat on both), but, as would later so often happen to worthy projects, this one languished when no implementing funds could be obtained from private foundations or from government.

Despite this setback, ASIM never wavered from its course of emphasizing the importance of the quality aspects of medical care. It was Ross Taylor who came up with the classic aphorism that the cost and quality of medical care are inseparable, and it was he who displayed the balance and dignity of the ASIM cause in his paper published in an issue of the ACP *Bulletin* in 1961, "ASIM—The First Five Years."

The quality of medical care—and its inseparability from cost—was given repeated emphasis by ASIM leaders in the early sixties. Successive presidents made the socio half of socio-economic a prominent part of their inaugural addresses, their speeches to component societies and other bodies, and their writings. Public relations chairmen, notably Malcolm Watts, hammered away at the point. Executive Director Bert Whitehall wrote on the subject in his column in *The Internist* and talked about it in his extensive travels around the country.

The 1967 Planning Committee report challenged ASIM to develop meaningful "standards" or "guidelines" of excellence in many aspects of health care, including office practice, hospital practice, continuing professional competence, and utilization of paramedical personnel. The 1970 planning report, while it included consideration of such issues as cost, financing and efficiency, placed as much or more emphasis on delivery systems, continuing education, manpower, technology and quality itself.

ASIM's emphasis on other than economic matters was by no means limited to rhetorical expressions of concern. Characteristically, the Society slowly but surely entered into a practical implementation and expression of its conceptual interest in the quality of care. What was to become at decade's end a broad tapestry of involvement in the field started out as a few small threads.

One thread, what might be called a research strand, consisted of the search for a method of assessing quality. The impetus came from an ASIM component which had forged ahead of the national Society in this arena. The New York State Society of Internal Medicine (NYSSIM) had enjoyed a string of able and aggressive leaders, including Virgil Beck, Herbert Berger, Charles Weller, Robert Schwinger and Robert Kohn. Notable among these pioneers was John Williams, who had already contributed his cinematic public relations skills in the film "Case History," which had done much to demonstrate to viewers exactly what an internist does.

By the early sixties, Williams had turned to a new interest, this time the possibility of assessing, through review of medical records, what doctors—naturally, internists—do in their office practices. The method of medical audit was beginning to gain credibility in the hospital setting, but conventional wisdom had it that the technique would not work in the office setting, where care elements and recordkeeping were both so strikingly different from those found in the hospital. Undaunted, Williams made contact with Cecil Sheps, PhD, noted health services researcher, who was also interested in the concept of office audit. The upshot was a study, jointly sponsored by the University of Pittsburgh and the NYSSIM, in which trained medical record analysts traveled to physicians' offices—volunteer internist-members of NYSSIM—to try to gather data from their records about the care they delivered. The results were interesting, if somewhat discouraging: It is possible to cull important data about patient care from the office records of internists, but the job is made very difficult—and to some degree inconclusive—because of deficiencies (in legibility and in content) in the way medical records are kept.

The study, despite its somewhat negative connotations, was a pioneering effort. It added luster—as Williams undoubtedly had foreseen—to the NYSSIM name, and, by association, to ASIM's name. An office quality audit subcommittee was added to the ASIM Council on Medical Services roster of committees and, not surprisingly, the person appointed to chair it was John Williams.

Its scope of interest expanded dramatically. By the late sixties, the committee had become the Quality Evaluation Committee of the Research and Development Council and its charge was "to develop, evaluate and recommend measures to assure the maintenance of high quality care by the internist."

At the time of the 1970 Annual Meeting in Philadelphia, word was received that DHEW's Center for Health Services Research had awarded a grant to ASIM (through its SEREF arm) to study the office care of internists, this time comparing patient care as culled from the records with pre-determined criteria for optimal care set by their peers. The study would take a couple of years to complete and when reported nationally in the early seventies, would also lend considerable prestige to the ASIM name.

Out of this study would come some of ASIM's major thrusts in the seventies—its development of the Assessment by Performance concept, its involvement in Private Initiative in PSRO and Private Initiative in Quality Assurance, and its championing of performance review as the best way of demonstrating professional accountability, in preference to passing recertification exams and giving evidence of participation in continuing medical education exercises.

A second thread in the tapestry of ASIM's quality thrust was its interest in the growing application of technology to the delivery of medical care.

In 1964, well before electronic data processing had captured the public's—or the profession's—fancy, ASIM devoted a major segment of its Annual Meeting program to a panel discussion about "the effect of computers on internal medicine." Program Chairman Sidney Krasnoff of Philadelphia, taking cognizance of his own early interest in the topic, delivered the first paper, entitled "Cybernetics—Medicine's Friend or Foe?" His preparatory research later grew into a 1967 book, *Computers in Medicine,* one of the first published on the subject.

Later, Charles Weller, an ASIM Trustee from New York, pursued the computer subject further, particularly as it applied to the medical record and the potential of data processing to store and retrieve information. Weller and Joseph Painter helped Irving Kanner, an ASIM member from Kentucky, pursue his interest in a simple method of applying computer technology to the office records of internists. Weller also made contact with the computer industry and struggled—fruitlessly it turned out—to see if IBM's complex project, the Clinical Decision Support System (CDSS), might have some usefulness for ASIM members.

Weller's contacts with technology experts led ASIM to establish relationships with other organizations, including the Society for Advanced Medical Systems, the Alliance for Engineering in Medicine and Biology, and the Association for Medical Instrumentation. Although some economy-minded Trustees were vocal in expressing skepticism about the value and cost-effectiveness of these relationships, there was no question about the fact that ASIM had established a place in the front line of medical technology. Later, William Felts became ASIM's computer champion and took advantage of his connection with the Control Data Corporation to keep ASIM Trustees abreast of the latest in EDP technology.

Another part of ASIM's technology thread dealt with the growing deployment of groups offering automated multiphasic health testing (AMHT) services. The prototype was Morris Collen's unit at the Kaiser-Permanente Clinic in Oakland, where he offered an array of testing services, some of it done by trained allied health personnel and some by technologic equipment. People coming through the unit could get nearly all of the services normally provided by an internist at a periodic physical examination—a history form to be filled out, much of a physical exam, x-ray studies, electrocardiograms, and a battery of laboratory tests. ASIM member Fred Gilbert, head of the AMHT center at the Straub Clinic in Honolulu, even reported the possible use of trained technicians to perform proctosigmoidoscopic exams. All of this, performed in assembly line fashion, with much contact with technology and technicians and little or no contact with a physician, could be delivered relatively cheaply—and, naturally, the data forthcoming could be stored in computers and retrieved for tabulation and display in elaborate printouts.

At one point in the late sixties AMHT centers were the rage, and there were seers who prophesied that they would shortly blanket the country. ASIM's response to this challenge was uncharacteristically ambivalent. On the one hand, the centers fulfilled some of ASIM's criteria of excellence: they were efficient (using both technology and allied health professionals), the data they produced were of uniformly high quality (except in a few fly-by-night commercial ventures), and their motives—early detection of disease and the accumulation over time of sound data on populations of patients—were hard to denigrate. On the other hand, the periodic evaluation of presumably well people was—cost-effective or not—the average internist's stock in trade. Besides which, a convincing argument could be made that AMHT units omitted the single most important element of the periodic examination—the personal contact between patient and physician, with its opportunity to dispel anxiety and to provide useful health education.

ASIM settled for monitoring the AMHT movement. A committee was appointed (first with Joseph Painter, later with William Felch as its chairman) within ASIM; it later joined with representatives from other interested professional organizations (such as the American College of Radiology and, especially, the College of American Pathologists) to establish the Interspecialty Society Committee for Multiphasic Health Screening. Guidelines were established for assuring the quality of AMHT and for what internists should do if they received a printout from an AMHT center about an individual who might or might not be a bona fide patient.

The flurry of interest in AMHT subsided by the early seventies, despite the assertions of Kaiser's Sidney Garfield that doctors were the bottleneck in the delivery of medical care and that the traffic flow would be eased if only all the "worried well" were triaged through the sieve of AMHTs. ASIM's committee and the Interspecialty Committee were disbanded. However, out of this flurry of activity grew ASIM's ongoing concern with the quality of office laboratory services, a concern that would lead in the seventies to its innovative Medical Laboratory Evaluation program.

Another thread in the technology skein was ASIM's new attention to manpower issues. The Carnegie Commission report of 1970 had asserted that a shortage existed in health manpower, both absolute and in terms of distribution by geography and by specialty—a shortage to which many harassed and overburdened ASIM members could attest.

One acclaimed solution was to produce a cadre of physician extenders trained to take over some of the tasks traditionally performed by doctors but not requiring their professional expertise.

ASIM entered this arena by taking advantage of a widely used information-securing instrument, the survey questionnaire. Employing the expert help of San Francisco statistician Maury Gershenson, the energy and intelligence of Trustee Frank Riddick (who had been ASIM's Young Internist of the Year in 1969), the solid and thoughtful advice of Addis Costello, chairman of the Practice Management Committee, and John Bryan, chairman of the Surveys Committee, ASIM in

1970 produced and distributed a questionnaire designed to elicit information about how internists use allied health personnel. The sample of 3,425 internists in 1,800 offices employed more than 8,500 full-time and part-time allied health workers. The data obtained showed that member-internists did make use of allied health workers, but with wide regional differences and with much divergence in what the respondents said they would like to delegate compared with what they actually did delegate. As far as providing solutions for the manpower shortage, the impact of conducting a survey may have been less than dramatic. But the survey results were published and received quite a bit of editorial comment. Once again, ASIM had proved to be at least in the thick of things and perhaps in the vanguard of new developments.

The final thread in the quality tapestry is captured by the phrase "peer review." From the beginning, ASIM had been in favor of doctors policing their own shop and against the notion that outsiders, especially nonprofessionals, should be involved. It had advised its members to get involved with health insurers to help resolve disputes, whether about the size of fees or the appropriateness of services rendered. And it had endorsed, without much fanfare, internists' efforts in their local hospitals to deal with the credentialling of and privilege delineation for their colleagues on the medical staff.

These postures were sporadic and unfocused until 1965, when the passage of the Medicare and Medicaid entitlements suddenly placed the federal government in the position of requiring the profession to embark on a program of utilization review—the evaluation of the appropriateness of the services rendered to program beneficiaries. ASIM's reaction was both prompt and thorough, and its task forces and committees quickly perceived a fundamental new force in the medical care firmament: a thrust toward a requirement for the profession to be accountable for its dealings with patients, to be responsible for assuring them about the cost, the quantity and—especially—the quality of their care.

This new demand for accountability was not likely to win instant popularity among doctors, particularly individualistic ones who cherished their independence and were wary of anyone—even colleagues—looking over their shoulders. But the times demanded its acknowledgment and ASIM responded with energy, not merely bowing to the inevitable but embracing the concept as a legitimate, even essential, component of professionalism. The technique of peer review—evaluation by one's equals—was just beginning to be explored in various settings in different parts of the country. ASIM's contribution was to grasp the idea and make of it a positive, uplifting professional symbol, its purpose educational rather than punitive. If this altruistic approach could be accepted and implemented by the profession, then the regulatory incursions of government might be fended off.

During the late sixties, the message was delivered to the ASIM membership, both directly in speeches and papers from the leadership and indirectly through a component society campaign. Conferences were held, lectures given, and symposia presented, all calculated to make the ASIM hierarchy understand the meaning and implications of quality. At one such symposium, at which noted health services researcher Paul Sanazaro was the featured speaker at the dais while the other panelists were seated behind him on a raised platform, one of the latter, ASIM Trustee Ben Hall, got so intrigued by the speaker's remarks that he shifted his chair a few inches—and fell off the platform (his colleagues later called it a "quality performance").

The rest of organized medicine was slower than ASIM to swallow the peer review bolus. To be sure, the College, under its able president (and articulate supporter of worthwhile ASIM campaigns), Washington State's James Haviland, had endorsed the concept. But the AMA, while paying lip service to the idea, had not put its full weight behind it, whether because some of its conservative elements were against the idea or because it was uncertain how to convert rhetoric to reality.

ASIM decided to put its hard-won credibility—and its modest political clout—to the test. It sought and was granted a meeting with the AMA Board. In November 1970, ASIM's Executive Committee—President Joseph Painter, Immediate Past President Clyde Greene, President-Elect Otto Page and Secretary-Treasurer Blaine Hibbard—along with Executive Director (and old AMA hand) William Ramsey—traveled to Boston and made its pitch to the AMA Board gathered there. They returned triumphant. AMA had agreed to cosponsor with ASIM a Peer Review Workshop designed to give attendees practical, how-to education about the mechanics of peer review. An ASIM committee—Joseph Painter, Charlotte Baer, William Felch—was assigned to work with their opposite numbers in the AMA to design the workshop agenda.

The conference was a resounding success. As the June 1971 *Internist* reported it, "some 400 of the nation's most knowledgeable practitioners assembled at the LaSalle Hotel in Chicago, May 21-22 for an AMA-ASIM cosponsored Workshop Conference on Peer Review. For the first time in the short history of peer review conferences, a workshop format allowed all the participants to learn with and from each other by reviewing some of the cases of practicing peer review committees."

Clearly, the AMA imprimatur—and its clout—were now solidly behind the peer review approach, both as an idea and as a method. And equally clearly, ASIM had been responsible for securing the support of the AMA. For the whole world to see, ASIM was the champion at the pinnacle of the peer review movement.

5

Coping with Legislation
Ambitious Assignment

ASIM's traditional concern for economic matters (reimbursement of internists' services) and its growing involvement in social aspects (accountability for the quality of care) could be conveniently combined under the heading of "socioeconomic(s)"—a word that was tirelessly repeated in ASIM pronouncements during the sixties. But a major part of ASIM's energy in this decade, particularly during its latter half, was devoted to a new concern. Its executive director in the early sixties, Bert Whitehall, writing in a column in The Internist, *made an attempt to insert this new aspect into the word by creating a new one: socio-politico-economic. But this didn't roll off the tongue too easily, and ASIM's leaders were forced to expand the word into a phrase: "The social, economic and political aspects. . ."*

It was not a sudden decision in 1965 to begin considering government incursions into the health care arena. The Society had had a Committee on Legislation from the beginning. For years, it had freely expressed opinions about proposed federal legislation, both in written form and occasionally as direct testimony before a congressional committee (as Stewart Seigle had done in 1961). And ASIM had long since established a strategic policy about legislative matters: it would apply its limited resources to trying to influence only those pieces of legislation that would clearly have an impact on or affect the care rendered by internists; the rest it would leave to the better-funded AMA to deal with. (This strategy was not always adhered to; for a while in the late sixties, ASIM got caught up in an enthusiasm to do battle with anti-vivisectionists and their proposed legislation to limit research involving animals.)

But the sixties saw increasing political emphasis on health matters. Each session of Congress explored the possibility of some form of national health insurance. (Wilbur Cohen, assistant secretary of DHEW, had discussed the topic as a speaker at ASIM's 1962 Annual Meeting in Philadelphia.) ASIM had supported the AMA in opposition to these proposals, which regularly ended up being bottled up in committee and not acted on by Congress as a whole.

But the election of 1964 brought an end to the indecision about a federal role in financing health care. When it became evident that some kind of legislation would pass, ASIM leaders, under President Malcolm Watts, decided it was time to get involved. The component societies were queried by telegram and the consensus was that ASIM should assume an active leadership role and work to achieve some kind of arrangement that would take into account the strong political thrust for some form of a national health care program, but one that would still permit practicing physicians to continue to give their patients high quality care.

ASIM's concerns were voiced at the AMA House of Delegates meeting in Miami Beach in late November, 1964 (ASIM's Board was meeting there at the same time). ASIM urged—directly and through the 46 ASIM members in the AMA House—that AMA reconsider its approach to the Kerr-Mills and the King-Anderson kinds of legislation. AMA reacted to this pressure appropriately, asking ASIM to submit constructive and detailed proposals for consideration by the AMA Council on Legislative Activities. Immediately thereafter, ASIM's Board met and, after intensive discussion, came up with a series of principles and propositions that were embodied in "A Proposal for the Accreditation of Health Care Plans and for a Federal Health Care Fund." Working with characteristic dispatch, ASIM had the proposal prepared and widely distributed by mid-December. On January 8, the proposal was presented to the AMA Council on Legislative Activities, and was received cordially and discussed in detail with some tangible support. But apparently, some political maneuvering had been going on behind the scenes at AMA: On January 9, AMA made public announcement of its "Eldercare" proposal.

But by this time ASIM had the bit in its teeth and was not ready to retreat from the scene. A survey was conducted which found, as had been suspected, that among the ASIM membership were internists who had close personal contact—often as personal physicians—with a majority of the members of the U.S. Senate. These contacts were put to use, with the result that ASIM was given the opportunity to present its case before the powerful Senate Finance Committee. Dr. Watts made the presentation in his usual scholarly but forceful manner, citing the position that ASIM, while it disapproved of the bill under consideration, believed that some legislation would be passed and wished to have it conform to ASIM principles as closely as possible. The hearing was respectful, although during the question-and-answer period after the prepared testimony had been delivered, Dr. Watts was asked some peppery questions by committee members.

The rest is history. Congress proceeded to amend the Social Security Law, adding Title 18 (Medicare), Title 19 (Medicaid) and Title 5 (maternal and infant health). One could cynically contend that ASIM's positions were totally submerged in the torrent of testimony and political infighting that shaped the final legislation. More optimistically, one could argue that ASIM's principles had exerted at least some small influence in determining the outcome of some of the provisions of the new Titles.

But some things are certain. ASIM had demonstrated its ability to develop rational, well thought-out positions on a complicated legislative subject. It had shown its willingness to stake out its positions within the framework of organized medicine and to win support for them there. And it had proven its capacity for getting its positions listened to in the congressional seats of power. To ASIM's clout in social and economic matters could now be added its clout in the political aspects of health care.

By March 1965, the legislative battle was over. Medicare and Medicaid were the law of the land. Now came their implementation, a bureaucratic, regulatory revolution that would have a profound effect on internists and their patients who were old and poor. Once again ASIM reacted forcefully, if anything displaying even more vigor than it had in the months before the law was passed.

The same month that Medicare was passed, Robert Westlake took over as ASIM's ninth president. Recognizing that his predecessor "already had the bit in his teeth," Westlake appointed Malcolm Watts to chair a task force charged with helping ASIM members to cope with the implementation of the new law. The members of the task force—James Feffer, William Felch, Frank Foster, Wendell Gordon, Clyde Greene, Malcolm Watts and Charles Weller—met promptly and devised an educational strategy, one which was quickly approved by the Board. Three separate regional meetings would be held for leaders from component societies. Workbooks containing summaries of the law and other appropriate materials would be prepared and handed out to attendees. Preliminary prepared talks would be delivered at the meetings: Watts for overview, Feffer for Medicare, Felch for Medicaid, etc. Question-and-answer periods would follow, after which participants would work in small group sessions to hammer out details and to make sure their understanding was sufficiently deep that they could go home and spread the word to their constituencies.

This plan required a remarkable logistical effort on the part of ASIM staff to make the arrangements for the meetings and to prepare the voluminous (and somehow frequently changing) workbooks. And, it required a remarkable commitment of time for preparation, travel and participation on the part of task force members.

Yet this remarkably vital organization—still less than ten years old—pulled it off. Within months after the passage of the Medicare/Medicaid law, ASIM got the word out—through its component society leaders to its rank-and-file members—about how to cope with the profound changes the law would impose on the practice of internal medicine.

While it is convenient to see this massive effort as a top-down dissemination strategy, flowing from the Board/Task Force out to the component leadership and finally to rank-and-file members, the fact is that ASIM's bottom-up flow also was at work. A good example is that of Charles Steele, Maine's down east cracker-barrel philosopher, who, seeing the difficulty his own over-65 patients were having in coping with Medicare red tape, single-handedly devised a couple of brochures to clarify its intricacies for them. He submitted these to ASIM, which after some editorial changes by an expert committee adopted the Steele brochure and offered it to the rest of the membership.

The Medicare/Medicaid legislation was by no means the only piece in the jigsaw puzzle of the Great Society. Many other pieces would also have an impact on internists and their patients. A notable example was the Heart, Cancer and Stroke proposals—also called the DeBakey bill after its principal proponent, the noted Texas vascular surgeon. Based on the notion that practitioners of medicine were not keeping abreast of rapidly developing scientific information, the legislation originally proposed setting up regional treatment centers to provide what later would be called tertiary care. After intense reaction from organized medicine, the legislation was watered down and the final version settled for funding two lesser alternatives, the Regional Medical Programs—to devise local initiatives for transmitting new information to practitioners—and the Comprehensive Health Planning Program—to coordinate local planning for health facilities and health care delivery.

ASIM, of course, had reacted promptly to the proposals. A Watts-drafted position paper was discussed, amended slightly, and approved by the ASIM Board as the Society's official position. Since it tended this time to coincide substantially with that of the AMA and the rest of organized medicine, there was no need to mount a major separate strategy to influence the course of legislative events. But when the final version of the bill was signed into law, ASIM recognized its potential impact on the practice of internal medicine. The result was that the traveling road show of 1965, while principally devoted to Medicare/Medicaid, also presented a detailed analysis of the RMP/CHP duo and recommendations for internists' response to them.

The passage of the Great Society legislation of the mid-sixties and ASIM's prompt reaction to it did not signal the end of ASIM's involvement with legislative matters (even though the Task Force was discharged and its purview returned to the normal council/committee structure). Although there was some slowdown in the passage of major legislation, there still remained the implementing regulations for internists to face. ASIM was better able than most professional organizations to understand the intricate usual-customary-reasonable fee concept and to do battle with bureaucratic attempts to conserve federal dollars by manipulating the fee mechanism.

But two major health care proposals involving legislation were standing by, waiting in the wings for the right moment to come on stage. One was national health insurance, sidetracked but not derailed by the passage of Medicare/Medicaid, and still touted vigorously by its ardent supporters as a necessary entitlement of the American people. The other was cost containment, the push to slow down the spiraling increase in health care costs.

By now, ASIM had developed a systematic approach for dealing with issues as they arose. In the case of NHI (ASIM incidentally preferred to use the phrase UHI—Universal Health Insurance—as connoting the same degree of entitlement but a lesser implication of nationalization), a set of principles was worked and reworked through committees, a definition of "comprehensive health care" was conjured up, and an ad hoc committee (presumably with the same narrow scope as, but a longer tenure than, a task force) to study legislative proposals and to offer suggestions for ASIM's posture.

In the case of cost containment, ASIM dealt with this newer and less focused topic with a broad brush: its fifteenth annual meeting program session was entitled, "The Internist and the Rising Cost of Medical Care" and dealt, conceptually and practically, with the causes of escalating costs and how internists could help contain them.

Forged in the crucible of the Great Society legislation of the mid-sixties, ASIM, by the time of its fifteenth birthday, was a finely honed instrument, ready to cope with the legislative and regulatory forces that it would face in the decade ahead.

6

Signs of Growth

Arguments, Almanacs, Anniversaries

ASIM's growth in the sixties could be measured not only in terms of major evolutionary changes, but also in a host of small increments: challenges met, crises averted, innovations begun—and some recurring tasks faced with studied effort.

In the decade of the sixties, relationships between the two sister organizations, ASIM and ACP, started and ended on a cordial basis. But in between, there were occasions when the placid flow was interrupted by patches of white water, eruptions of turbulent emotions and ruffled feelings.

Back in 1957, ASIM had invited the College to send observers to ASIM Board meetings so that the College could always keep abreast of what was going on in the Society's chambers. By 1959, the mechanism had become a formal one, and three College representatives formed an official ACP Liaison Committee charged with attending ASIM meetings. The mechanism, albeit somewhat unidirectional, seemed to work reasonably well, at least up until 1963. In September of that year, ACP President Wesley Spink announced at the Southeastern Regional Meeting of the College that ACP intended to become active in the socioeconomic aspects of internal medicine. In November, the ACP Board of Regents, meeting with the executive committee of the Board of Governors, formally changed the status quo by creating a Committee on Medical Services.

ASIM, through President Maxwell Berry, promptly complained about the College's new tack, and later backed up that complaint with a poll of ASIM members (most of whom were also College members) which revealed that an overwhelming majority wanted the Society to "continue to pursue vigorously its established policy of representing internists in the area of socioeconomics and related fields." As always in such conflicts, there was much misunderstanding about and misinterpretation of the exact nature of the contretemps.

In April 1964, Malcolm Watts became ASIM's new president, and the College's new president, Thomas M. Durant, was more sympathetic to ASIM's separate mission than his predecessor had been. Saying "let us be on with the job," Watts appointed an ad hoc liaison committee to meet with ACP representatives. At the first joint liaison meeting in June 1964, the 15 individuals in attendance agreed that cooperation between the two organizations should become the established mode, set up principles delineating the province of each, and recommended that regular liaison be carried out thereafter.

Harmony, or at least the lack of discord, prevailed thereafter for nearly five years. But in 1968, the pot began to boil again. The College, as many of its Regents' meetings seemed to indicate, was once again examining its posture vis-à-vis socioeconomics and was speculating about the possibility of seeking some amalgamation of the two organizations. Clearly, the issues were too weighty for anything but top-level liaison. ASIM President James Feffer, working closely with his opposite number in the College, Rudolph Kampmeier, sought a joint meeting of the policy-making leadership of both organizations.

This was agreed to by both Boards, and in April 1968, the meeting took place, with consensus decisions arrived at by the ten participants (for ASIM Feffer, Long, Gordon, Hibbard and Painter; for the College Kampmeier, Pollard, Wright, Haviland and Smith). The result is called the Phoenix Accord (that the meeting was held in Scottsdale is a minor historical inaccuracy) which spelled out in unequivocal terms the separate turf of the two organizations:

> "In recognition of the desirability of closer liaison between the American College of Physicians and the American Society of Internal Medicine, a new liaison committee has been established to represent the top policy level of both organizations. This committee consists of the president, president-elect, and immediate past president of each, two ACP Regents and two ASIM Trustees. The first meeting was held in Phoenix, Arizona on February 4 and 5, 1968.
>
> "The committee recognized and reaffirmed unanimously the distinct need for two separate organizations: The American College of Physicians primarily in consideration and evaluation of medical and scientific knowledge and in medical education; The American Society of Internal Medicine primarily in consideration and evaluation of the socioeconomic aspects of the practice of medicine and their application to the delivery of health services. The committee agreed there are also areas of mutual responsibility in the provision of the best possible medical care.
>
> "This committee acknowledged that each organization must be sensitive to activities and programs of the other. Therefore, it recognized the need for closer cooperation involving areas of common interest. Subsequent meetings will seek to identify those areas and to develop methods for effective action."

Top level liaison continued for some years thereafter. Out of it grew the mechanisms for internal medicine's participation in AMA affairs, through joint membership on the Interspecialty Advisory Board and through combined involvement in the Section Council of Internal Medicine. The key tactic was alternation, in voice and vote for the IAB and in status as delegate or alternate delegate for internal medicine's single vote in the AMA House of Delegates. The key strategy was to reach consensus positions ahead of time so as to present a common front for internal medicine. The key mode was one of cooperation. Out of this mode would come two events: the unsuccessful 1972 attempt at a merger and, in 1976, the successful creation of the Federated Council for Internal Medicine.

In the early sixties, the Society's principal means of communicating with its members was the *ASIM Newsletter,* a brief summary of Society activities, national and component, published at the energetic rate of ten times a year (although some thought that six fatter issues would be preferable). The publication was under the aegis of the Public Relations Committee; its early sixties chairman, Malcolm Watts, was thus the first de facto editor and his fine editorial hand can be seen in his periodic columns and in the make-up and style of the fledgling communications medium. The newsletter contained, among other features, a regular column by Executive Director Whitehall, and a less-than-regular column by the current president.

By 1963, despite the fact that its official name had become *The Internist,* the publication's format was still that of a newsletter and ASIM leaders were casting about for ways and means of making it a more effective instrument. One route that was studied was to change to a full-fledged journal, one that would publish scientific papers about socioeconomic matters. This notion was turned down on the grounds of expense and editorial difficulties (although at decade's end the possibility of ASIM's sponsoring a socioeconomic section in the *American Journal of Medicine* was studied—and again turned down).

The alternative seemed clear. *The Internist* needed an editor and in June 1964, President Watts announced the appointment of Joseph Furlong of San Francisco to that position. Later, an editorial advisory board was appointed to assist him, consisting of Richard Bates, John Berry, Fred Bulter, R. Brian Grinnan, John Marietta, Peter Talso and Edwin Evans. The new editor was invited to attend Board meetings to assure that he grasped the flavor as well as the official substance of its actions. Under his leadership, *The Internist* became a different and more effective medium for communicating with Society members.

Its masthead was distinctive and its black on green, Old English lettering was readily recognizable (to the degree that Frank Foster made the classic, if ambiguous, remark, "It reminds me of something I would expect in church."). The frequency of publication was cut back to six issues a year, but the number of pages per issue increased substantially, and later during Furlong's stewardship the number of issues grew to 12 a year. The content changed impressively too: There was still much news of ASIM activities—who said what at which meeting, but there was increasing evidence of philosophical and conceptual content, often clustered in themes, explaining the why as well as the what of Society activities.

ASIM, though less than 15 years old in 1970, was even then proud of its history; Furlong arranged for a year-by-year series of "Past Problems and Their Solutions," each offered by a past president who outlined the principal events of his administration and interpreted their significance and impact. Furlong served as editor under seven ASIM presidents. In submitting his resignation, he reported that during his tenure, *The Internist* had grown from an annual output of six issues with a total of 24 pages in 1964 to 12 issues with 162 pages in 1970. He was succeeded in 1971 by Clyde Greene, who had just completed his tour as immediate past president, and who would continue as editor until 1975.

During the sixties, the Society's growth was also demonstrated in terms of its supporting staff. In 1967, it was decided that a different and broader set of management skills was needed to back up the increasingly complex activities being carried out by the ASIM leadership.

There was talk of looking for an internist who also had administrative skills; Clyde Greene's name was mentioned again. But eventually the conclusion was reached that the Society would be better off to preserve the separation of powers between the elected leadership and paid staff; a non-physician exec was indicated.

After a thorough search, the ASIM leaders came up with a first-class candidate. William R. Ramsey was young and possessed the vigor and enthusiasm of youth. He was also experienced, having served in the ranks of organized medicine for some years, most recently with the AMA's field service staff which made contact with state medical associations and specialty societies. And his letters of recommendation mentioned desirable qualities: intelligence, reliability, thoroughness, and devotion to duty.

In 1968, Bill Ramsey was hired. He joined a small staff—only he and Dorothy Titland remain today of that original cadre. It is sufficient to say that during the 13 intervening years Bill Ramsey has presided over the growth and development of a staff that is today second to none.

An easily visible and regularly recurring signpost of ASIM's growth and development during the sixties was its annual meeting. Held in the spring of the year (ranging from late March to early May, nearly always just before the ACP's annual meeting) and in a variety of locations (including Philadelphia, Denver, Atlantic City, Chicago, New York, San Francisco, Boston), the annual meetings marked the occasion for the ASIM family to take up matters of policy, both conceptually—in the selection of program session topics and speakers—and practically—in the consideration of reports, recommendations and resolutions by the House of Delegates.

The choice of topics during the sixties reveals an interesting mixture of concerns. In 1962, the then-new subject of quality of care (and its inseparability from economics) was featured, with speakers representing hospitals, medical schools, the pharmaceutical industry, government (even then it was Wilbur Cohen, talking about health insurance for the aged), the Blues, labor, and internal medicine (represented by Florida's Jere Annis who, in 1973, would be ASIM's Distinguished Internist). In 1963 the topic was global ("Internal Medicine and Its Future"), with speakers promoting the general internist, multi-specialty groups, single-specialty groups and solo practice; a second session presented forces influencing the practice of internal medicine, such as prepaid group practice, medical care foundations, and government. The 1964 program introduced a session on the influence of medical schools and medical centers on the practice of internal medicine, followed by a second session on the brand new subject of computers in medicine.

In 1965, the subject matter turned to practical matters, with discussants talking about "This Is Your Practice." The 10th Annual Meeting in 1966 focused on "Utilization . . . Medical Judgment," discussing utilization of diagnostic and therapeutic tools, and ending with a talk about the then-new arena of utilization review under Medicare. In 1967, the focus once again was on change, both in public expectations (as seen by management and labor) and in patterns of medical care (community health and—for the first time—use of physician extenders). The next year highlighted physician attitudes and behavior patterns, the two principal sessions being "Motivation In Medicine" and "The Efficient Internist." The 1969 list was a potpourri ranging from the global ("Can the Traditional Practice of Medicine Survive?") to the professional ("The Crisis in Medical Education") to the practical ("Trends in Income Arrangements"). In 1970, the much debated question of access to care was presented, with one panel devoted to "Health Care for the Disadvantaged," the other to "Health Care for the 'Middle American.'" For its fifteenth meeting, in 1971, ASIM chose to talk about the subject that would become the principal health care issue of the decade: "The Internist and the Rising Costs of Medical Care."

The annual meetings had other program elements aside from the formal sessions. There were luncheon speakers, frequently the President of the College or of the AMA, at times the current Surgeon General or Assistant Secretary of Health for HEW, perhaps an FDA Commissioner or a director of the NIH. Then there were banquets, usually black-tie affairs, with distinguished speakers from public life, their subject matter ranging from the humorous (columnist Bob Considine), through the earnest (*Christian Science Monitor* editor Edwin Canham), to the scientific (Dr. Charles Berry of NASA). There was room at the meetings for the sentimental (awards to distinguished internists, such as Dwight Wilbur, Wallace Yater, Roberta Fenlon), the inspirational (awards to young internists—Frank Riddick, Alfred Biggs, Joseph Katterhagen), and the laudatory (commendations for service to ASIM—John Williams, Joseph Furlong, Robert Raborn, Clyde Greene).

Annual meetings also had time for some fun: enjoying the host city, cocktail parties (some sponsored, some "no-host"), entertainment (the Princeton Nassoons singing group), and late-night relaxation (dancing, after the formal speeches were finally over).

Attendees at annual meetings, it is clear, were both instructed and entertained. But most of them, the delegates from component societies, were there to take part in the politics of establishing policy for the growing Society.

In 1962, ASIM had 48 more-or-less active components. Not all of them sent delegates to the annual meeting in Philadelphia; 65 delegates representing 32 components did attend and participated in the deliberations of the policy-making House. The secretary-treasurer reported that $20 dues from 7,890 members was sufficient to approve a budget of $157,800 encompassing such things as the move to larger headquarters at 3410 Geary Boulevard in San Francisco, the hiring of executive director Whitehall, and a host of other money-consuming activities. The 1962 House also heard reports from the other officers and from a handful of standing committees, and considered 17 resolutions on a range of topics, including legislative activity, advertising in the *ASIM Newsletter,* annual physicals, and inter-specialty liaison.

In 1971, the picture was different. One hundred six delegates were seated after approval by the Credentials Committee, representing 48 of ASIM's 50 components. The House met in two sessions, with five reference committees hearing testimony in between. Reports were heard from the secretary-treasurer and the Finance Committee indicating the need for a dues structure of $70. The question of the establishment of a socio-economic journal was again reviewed. Following Dr. Painter's presidential address, 22 special reports of the Board of Trustees, reports of officers, councils and committees, and 22 resolutions, two introduced by the Board of Trustees and 20 by 12 component societies, were referred to the five reference committees. Resolutions that were approved dealt with Bylaws amendments (making all categories of component society members also members of ASIM); compensation for all necessary services, including concurrent care; the right of physicians to accept or reject Medicare assignment; reaffirmation of policy that physicians be urged to use direct billing; urging component societies to establish legislative committees; reaffirming ASIM policy to use non-governmental fiscal intermediaries in Medicaid; urging the ABIM to give equal weight to additional training in general internal medicine; asking ASIM to seek representation on the ABIM; asking ASIM to study the report of the Carnegie Commission on Higher Education; and urging all component societies to undertake immediately an intensive membership campaign.

Afterthought

It is a truism that most 15-year-olds live in no man's land, between childhood and adulthood, swinging from one to the other and back under a host of powerful external and internal forces.

Not so this ASIM teenager. It had made the switch to adulthood in a remarkably short period of time. By its 15th birthday in 1971, its voice had changed to one of resonant maturity and was listened to respectfully in health circles. It no longer had to beg for the attention of respected elders; instead, its opinions and positions were sought in their councils.

It had grown in size, so that by 1971 it was the fourth largest specialty society as measured by number of members. It had set out for itself a unique mission—to understand and to influence the social, economic and political aspects of health care. And it had proven—by measurable performance—its ability to carry out its objectives in an orderly and rational manner that made long-time observers of the health care scene marvel.

By 1971, ASIM had grown to maturity. The Society and its leaders could face the future with an adult self-confidence. No matter what problems or opportunities would arise in the decade ahead, this remarkable organization would be mature enough to cope with them effectively.

VOLUME III

The Mature Years

Adulthood and Authority

Aphorism: Maturity

Just as it would be laughable to assert that human beings change abruptly from the turmoil of adolescence to the comparative orderliness of adulthood, so would it be absurd to claim that ASIM changed overnight from a phase of growth to a phase of maturity. The truth, of course, is that the Society's growth and development, from 1956 to the present, can more accurately be viewed as a straight and—happily—upward-tilting line, than as a series of steps.

Still, ASIM's decade of the seventies did differ in many ways from the decade of the sixties, and it is possible, looking from a 1981 vantage point, to pick out a number of salient characteristics—both attitudinal and operational—that sharply distinguish one era from the other.

Just as adolescence is accompanied by a lack of self-confidence, so ASIM, in its growing years, was not always sure of its place in the scheme of things. Like most youngsters, it longed for—and sometimes battled for—a place in the sun. It was often introspective, calling planning sessions no less than three times in a decade and shifting its internal council/committee structure around in the hope that its function would be more efficient—and less awkward. When it turned to the external world, its aspiration was to achieve recognition, and it worked to achieve this end by asking members of the top echelons of the health enterprise to speak formally at its program sessions and to chat informally at its President-Elect's Advisory Council meetings. Seeking to be acknowledged, the Society leaders went around knocking on doors, asking to let its voice be heard, in such forums as the AMA and the ABIM. A key strategy was encompassed by the word liaison, signifying the desire to have contact with the major agencies in the health arena.

Happily, like the occasional adolescent who sails through the growing years a triumphant winner, ASIM managed during the sixties to achieve nearly all of the ends it yearned for. By the early seventies, the Society had indeed found its place in the sun.

Almost suddenly, it seemed, ASIM was a force to be reckoned with, an insider instead of an outsider, an important gear in the health engine. In its now less frequent introspective moments, it was motivated not by anxiety but by rationality, a cool, analytical review of goals, objectives, strategies and priorities. No longer the supplicant knocking on doors, ASIM had now become the target of supplications by others. The Society's leaders were no less busy than their predecessors, but instead of pressing to establish liaison relationships, they were now occupied in choosing which speaking engagement to accept and in selecting which multi-disciplinary advisory board or task force to serve on in order to further the interest of internists and their patients. And only a mature organization, confident of its destiny, would have the courage to pull up its roots and transplant them 3,000 miles to unfamiliar soil.

The grown-up ASIM of 1981 is a different organization than it was in the fifties and sixties. Today, its identity is firm, its goals spelled out, its role unambiguous, its image clear. And it was during the seventies that ASIM grew up.

1

Intraspecialty Relationships
Amalgamation or Alliance

During the seventies, ASIM expanded and sharpened its relationships with the rest of what is called (with some audacity) "organized" medicine. The strategy consisted in part of penetration—gaining access to the committees and councils of the AMA. Partly it was made up of paternalism—helping smaller subspecialty societies learn how to cope with the complex scene. Partly, it was plain liaison—meeting with other broad specialty organizations and deciding when to agree (to pursue some joint action) and when to disagree (so as to avoid overt conflict).

But with all this attention to the interests of the other layers of the multi-level structure of organized medicine, ASIM still made sure to take heed of its own principal concern: the needs of internists and their patients. Its major efforts, without any question, were within the structure of organized internal medicine.

A major event of the early seventies was an attempt—one that came within a hairsbreadth of consummation—to join the two major internist organizations into one.

The idea came up almost casually. Ever since the Phoenix Accord of 1968, the top elected leadership of ASIM and ACP had met together regularly, usually twice a year, as a formal Liaison Committee to discuss matters of mutual interest. Out of its deliberations came the successful mechanism for representing internists in the AMA, through the Section Council on Internal Medicine. Agreement had been reached on a number of other joint positions and actions as well.

It was in this climate of cooperation, that, at the June 1971, regular meeting of the Liaison Committee, an item appeared on the agenda called "The Future of Internal Medicine." The possibility was raised—cautiously—of merging the two organizations, and agreement was reached—gingerly—to have discussions about how such an amalgamation might be accomplished. It was also agreed that such discussions—since there was a distinct possibility that they might be broken off at an early stage—would be carried out secretly in the beginning in order to prevent the raising of false expectations and to avoid a hubbub of reaction from rank-and-file members.

The advantages of such a merger were clear: Internal medicine would be represented by a single voice, for both its biomedical and its socioeconomic thrusts. And the voice would have clout. ACP's 20,000 members and ASIM's 12,000 (with roughly 7,000 in common) would make the new body the fourth largest professional organization in the country—after the AMA, the American Academy of Family Physicians and the American College of Surgeons. The hurdles to be overcome were also obvious, including major problems like the differences in the structure and power flow of the two organizations, and minor ones like membership categories, dues structure, the location of a headquarters office, and the name of the new body. It was decided that each side would consider these and other issues, and would return to a meeting of the full Committee in September 1971 with some proposals.

The ASIM members of the committee—President Page, Past President Painter, President-Elect Evans, Secretary-Treasurer Hibbard and Trustee Felch—met several times during the summer, exploring the potential ramifications of amalgamation. They reached agreement that the technical matters of name, dues and location were solvable through negotiations. But they felt strongly that the principal question of structure and function of the new organization could only be resolved if it were to retain ASIM's grassroots flow of power, with state components making up a federation that would decide national policy.

At the September full Committee meeting the ASIM group found their ACP counterparts (President Butt, Past President Haviland, President-Elect Sodeman, Regent Berry and Governor Gamble) in surprising accord about the worthwhileness of state "chapters" and of the federation concept, including the right of a national house of delegates (they preferred to call it a "council") to set policy and to elect the national governing body ("board of directors"). The state "governors" could be elected by their constituent membership, would conduct local affairs, and be part of the national policy-making body. Not surprisingly, the ACP representatives wanted to preserve some of the cherished, fifty-year-old traditions of the College, including its name, so that its respected place in the professional firmament would not be lost.

There being no major disagreements, the members of the Liaison Committee decided—the mood shifting from tentativeness to commitment and beginning hope—to continue to hammer out the details. More meetings were held. Although both governing boards were, of course, apprised of the negotiations and, naturally, top staff was as well, the meetings were still held in secret since there was always the chance that an unanticipated snag could abort the whole effort. Accommodations were reached: instead of a new name, why not simply call the new organization ACP/ASIM? (A little cumbersome, but the AFL-CIO had managed to accept a similar compromise.) The lawyers were called in to determine what changes would be required in charters and bylaws and, finally, to draft a Memorandum of Intent. The headquarters office, despite some sentimental favor for San Francisco and some political opinion for Washington, D.C., might better be in Philadelphia where ACP had a sizable—and fully paid-for—building.

Finally, both Boards approved the decision to submit the Memorandum of Intent to the 1972 meetings of the policy-making bodies of the two organizations, ASIM's House of Delegates which would meet on April 14 and 16, and ACP's Boards of Governors and Regents which would meet on April 15 and 16—both in Atlantic City at headquarters hotels a few blocks apart.

A transcript has been preserved of the momentous hearing of ASIM's Reference Committee D (Oregon's Jules Bittner, chairman, Colorado's Jerry Appelbaum, Pennsylvania's David Feinberg, New York's Monte Malach and Louisiana's George Pankey) on April 15. Most of the testimony is in the vein of "I'm in favor of amalgamation, but—." To be sure, there are a few outspoken opponents, including prestigious past presidents, but these are balanced by some strong proponents willing to give unequivocal support to the Liaison Committee and the Board. A number of speakers express irritation with the preceding secrecy and the short, one month, interval between the announcement and the decision-making time—and the resultant inability to discuss the proposal with the "troops back home." Some humor shows up: Texan Jay Welch offers an alternative to marriage, "Why don't we just shack up with them?"

Predictably, much testimony is offered about pesky details. Voices are raised in favor of the "American College of Medicine" as a less cumbersome name. Philadelphia is denigrated, the preferred sites generally being San Francisco, Chicago, or, especially, Washington. Parliamentary buffs are wary about one provision limiting the terms of office of delegates/councillors and another provision requiring the future house/council to have a two-thirds instead of a simple majority to overrule decisions of the Board. The Liaison Committee members and other Trustees avoid the fray (except to clarify details), aware that people involved in negotiations tend to support the product of those negotiations and sensitive to the need for the House to make the decision without pressure. Dr. Butt, leader of the College, comes in and makes a few remarks (he has evidently been the "butt" of some critical remarks from parts of his camp) generally supporting the amalgamation but stressing the hallowed traditions of the College. The debate finally ends after nearly two hours, with the mood being generally pro-amalgamation.

Next day, Reference Committee D issued its report, in general supporting the amalgamation, but proposing strict amendments to the Memorandum of Intent omitting reference to Philadelphia and urging Washington, D.C., as the new organization's site, giving the house/council simple majority overrule power, and deleting reference to the terms of councillors.

A few blocks away, the College was having its problems. Some members of its Board of Governors, a body having significant advisory input to the Regents but no decision-making powers, were unhappy that they had been left in the dark until a month before. And there were reports—among the many rumors circulating that weekend—that some Regents were digging their heels in, fearful that the structure imposed by the amalgamation design would mean ASIM swallowing ACP.

Within 24 hours, the whole house of cards collapsed. To this day there are arguments about which organization said "no" first. Did one group, hearing reports of some of the negative opinions and positions of the other, decide first to vote the proposal down, with the other promptly following suit? Neither side particularly wanted to be portrayed publicly as the body primarily responsible for turning down a proposition that had attracted such widespread support. The fact is that by Sunday afternoon, both sides had decided that amalgamation was not viable.

Reaction to the decision was mixed. Feelings of being let down, of disappointment, even anger, were voiced, especially at having come so close to consummation after those long months of careful and thoughtful effort. So were expressions of relief, with philosophers asserting that the marriage would never have worked anyhow and pragmatists giving grateful thanks at not having to face months of further complex negotiations about details.

In any event, life would go on; the return to the status quo ante would have to be announced. Representatives met and a joint statement was drafted for transmission to both memberships, stating in part "while there was general approval of the concept of establishing a single new organization for internal medicine, there are fundamental differences in the authority for establishing policy and the methods of operation which preclude amalgamation at this time."

Amalgamation, for the foreseeable future, was dead.

One wonders if feelings of relief at failure of amalgamation may have been more prevalent, on both sides, than was publicly acknowledged. Certainly, there were no visible evidences of rancor or antagonism from either party. The top brass settled down into the previous leisurely practice of meeting once or twice a year to consider joint reactions to AMA resolutions and other matters of mutual interest. Disagreements were unusual and consensus the rule.

But apparently, there still lingered some worry about the lack of a common voice for internal medicine. The need for such a voice became especially urgent in the mid-seventies when alarm began to be voiced about the increasing trend to subspecialization. Suddenly, the virtues of primary care were being widely proclaimed; everyone rushed to get into the act, trying to work out a precise definition of primary care, to figure ways of getting future practitioners to consider it as a career choice, and to decide how best to teach it. Clearly, this was a topic of considerable importance to internal medicine, which, more than other disciplines, offered future physicians the options of a career in primary or subspecialty care—or, for that matter, both. Equally clearly, the topic was one which touched all facets of internal medicine—its medical school professors, its certifying board, its continuing educators, and its practitioners.

In 1974, the notion was explored of getting the organizations representing these elements within internal medicine—the Association of Professors of Medicine (APM), the American Board of Internal Medicine (ABIM), the ACP, and ASIM—to join together to establish policy and positions about the primary care issue and other major arenas of importance to internists. After some preliminary discussions to establish ground rules—a rotating chairmanship and secretariat, unanimous approval on all decisions (each organization thus having veto power)—the Federated Council for Internal Medicine (the acronym, FCIM, is pronounced "Fickum") was created, at least on the drawing board. The ASIM Board, in February 1975, approved in principle the Society's becoming a member, and appointed Secretary-Treasurer William Daines, Trustee Ben Hall and President-Elect Ralph Reinfrank as its first representatives. At that June's meeting of the House of Delegates, considerable negative sentiment was voiced, the principal argument being the old town-gown contention that the voice of the practicing internist (ASIM's) would be drowned out by the academicians in the other three organizations. But the right of veto was reassuring and the House finally endorsed entry into FCIM with only a sprinkling of negative votes.

In its first year, the new federation, after completing start-up administrative chores of establishing a charter, bylaws and procedural rules, tackled the primary care issue. ASIM, naturally, had for some time had a task force devoted to the subject and had developed a position paper. So had the ABIM. Evidence of willingness to compromise and negotiate was shown, especially on the part of FCIM's first-year chairman, ACP's able president Robert Petersdorf, and the APM's talented and equable Saul Farber (who two years later would be honored for his efforts in FCIM and in other arenas as ASIM's Distinguished Internist of the Year). After much interchange of paper, a joint position on primary care was achieved and disseminated.

By 1976, when ASIM's Ben Hall took over FCIM's chairmanship, he reported that the FCIM members had successfully gotten through the necessary group dynamics (he called it "de-mythologizing" each other) and had developed an agenda of some size, including jointly sponsoring a National Study of Internal Medicine Manpower (NaSIMM), appointing task forces devoted to increasing residency training slots in internal medicine, and organizing the directors of medical residency programs.

In the ensuing years, FCIM has continued to meet at regular intervals. New individuals have served as representatives from the member organizations; for ASIM, its spokesmen have been Carmault Jackson, William Millhon, Lonnie Bristow, Reggie Harris, Burns Roehrig, and, especially, Monte Malach, who chaired the ASIM delegation for several years and, in 1980, was FCIM's chairman.

How has FCIM worked out? It has successfully shown that a "single voice" for internal medicine can be displayed to the health care world, that policy positions can be hammered out (with much hard work) which represent the aggregate feelings of the four member organizations (five, if one now counts the input of the program directors). The veto has had little or no use; the representatives back away from trying to reach consensus when they perceive firm differences of opinion. Some worthwhile projects (e.g., the manpower study) have been carried out, and some useful positions reached which have influenced policy and implementation strategies, both within internal medicine and elsewhere. Most of all, FCIM has shown that internists coming from different backgrounds, having different perceptions of the real world, and representing different subsets of internal medicine, can come together and talk and educate each other. The benefits of such contact, though hard to quantify, are considerable.

The agenda of FCIM, by its nature, must be a sparse one, limited to the few policy issues that touch all segments of internal medicine. It follows that each member organization has a much larger agenda of its own, policies, programs and projects that are designed to advance its own interests within internal medicine.

By the late seventies, it was becoming clear that the ten-year-old Phoenix Accord, with its clear separation of powers between ASIM and ACP, could no longer work in the increasingly complex health care world. In 1977, the College and its new EVP, Robert Moser, were giving clear signals of their intention to plug into the social, economic, and political fronts. To accomplish this, the College announced its aim to form state chapters (which, for many ASIM component societies, would be direct competitors). And ASIM, with its push toward assessment of performance, was inevitably dealing with the scientific content of care. Signs of strain between the two organizations could be detected. The formal liaison (which had gradually dwindled into perfunctory and non-substantive contact) could not be expected to find a happy formula for an agreeable relationship.

Some ASIM spokesmen took a recriminatory stance. The College, they argued, had two decades earlier caused the creation of ASIM by its unwillingness to be concerned with social, economic, and political matters. And the College, which over the years had professed its desire to stick to the educational game and leave other matters to ASIM experts, now was invading the Society's turf.

But hurt feelings—in some minds a sense of betrayal—could not change the reality of the ACP's new tack. The answer for ASIM, its leadership concluded, was to continue to do its own thing and to do it exceedingly well. ASIM President William Daines outlined this position in a September 1977 *Internist* interview. First citing the Society's 20-year history of gradually increasing expertise and clout in its chosen arena of activity, next pointing out the strength of its federation structure, then listing its broad current agenda of ongoing and unfinished tasks, he went on to dispel any speculation that FCIM or another try at amalgamation could solve the problem. He expressed the hope that the College and the Society would keep in contact and try as much as possible not to present divergent views to the outside world. He finished by saying, "I am convinced that it is the activities of the Society and its components over the last 20 years that have been largely responsible for the recognition and stature of the practicing internist. My view—and it is supported by my fellow Trustees—is that we should continue our efforts to represent internists as effectively as possible in matters related to the practice of internal medicine. We welcome the support of all internists in carrying out this mission."

Today, in ASIM's 25th year, this "separate, but equal" doctrine still obtains. There is no visible evidence of friction, let alone hostility, between the two major organizations in internal medicine. They touch base with each other, particularly in such settings as meetings of the AMA House. There, they usually concur on positions; occasionally, they agree to disagree, as happened with a complex issue about chiropractic and with a debate as to whether housestaff members are students or employees or both. They are able to work together, as evidenced by their joint participation in FCIM and by their interlocking efforts in co-sponsoring the current Private Initiative in Quality Assurance project.

But, separate they are—and will continue to be for the foreseeable future. The College is presently in a start-up posture: It is opening a Washington office, it is charging its committees to discuss social, economic and political issues, and it is apparently committed to striving to forge a stronger local base through the creation of state chapters.

Meanwhile, ASIM goes about its business in its usual way, detecting issues of importance to internists and their patients, putting them through the analytical process of its task forces and committees, resynthesizing them into positions through the workings of the Board and the House, developing positions about them, and then devising and implementing strategies for educating internists about the issues and influencing others to make change.

2

Inside ASIM

Array of Activities

As ASIM matured, its self-confidence waxed and its compulsion for introspection waned. The evidence: It held only two formal planning sessions during the seventies, one in 1972 and one in 1976—and none since then. Nonetheless, the Society did continue to pay steady attention to its internal affairs and was constantly devising new ways to meet the needs of its constituents. And the principal means of communication with them, The Internist, *became an increasingly sophisticated publication, a mirror for ASIM's growing self-confidence.*

The first planning session of the seventies was held in the salubrious climate of Mexico. The trip to Acapulco, it turned out, was not that much more expensive than to a resort area in the U.S. Anyway, the attendees—12 Trustees, two Trustee nominees, a recent past president, an editor and two staff members—paid the difference themselves. The subject matter was not all that different from previous planning sessions: to relate the activities of ASIM to its environment, in this case, to three targets—the public, the internist, and other forces. Out of three half-days of discussion (some non-working time was allotted to seeing the sights) came nine long-term goals for ASIM activity and 15 specific recommendations on strategy.

Three Trustees (Felch, Felts, Riddick) and two staff persons (Ramsey, Titland) stayed on for a half-day to wrap up the loose ends and engage in the process of converting concepts to words. It seemed appropriate to combine this semantic fishing expedition with a real one, so a charter boat was hired. It is probably a tribute to the subcommittee's devotion to duty that a half hour's interruption, while Frank Riddick hooked and boated a 127-pound sailfish, was followed by a prompt return to the task at hand.

The second planning session in 1976 followed the tradition of being held in a resort area. But this time, perhaps in deference to the health care world's prevailing cost containment mood, it was held in home-base California, in luxurious Newport Beach. The focus this time around was less on outside environmental targets and more on ASIM itself, specifically its management process and how its limited resources might best be channeled to achieve (in the vernacular of the day) the biggest bang for the buck. The emphasis was less on structure (no simple reshuffling of Council and committee names would do as it had in the past) and more on function. ASIM's goal in life, its raison d'être, was hammered out first: "To achieve continued improvement of patient care." Its secondary goal came next: "To promote the continued growth and enhancement of the discipline of internal medicine and its practice, by assisting and supporting internists in their efforts to function optimally within an increasingly complex environment." Next came the identification of ASIM's principal objectives:

I. To be an advocate of the patient.
II. To increase the effectiveness of the internist.
III. To increase the efficiency of the internist.
IV. To protect the territory of the internist.
V. To improve the practice environment of the internist.
VI. To continue to increase the growth, strength, and effectiveness of ASIM.

For each of these six objectives a series of subobjectives was identified, each representing a major thread in the tapestry of ASIM activity. The finished product sounds straightforward enough, and the orderly list of objectives and subobjectives continues today to be the template against which ASIM programs are designed and evaluated. But their apparent simplicity is deceptive. They were achieved painfully, with much argument about nuances of meaning and with much disagreement (for instance, about the differences between subobjectives and strategies), all of which had to be ironed out before the final version was approved. But in the end, it was achieved. And henceforth, each ASIM activity would be assigned to an objective, each proposal for a new program would be checked to see how well it matched the template, and, at subsequent Board meetings, reports of completed work would be evaluated (by a Trustee assigned to that specific task) as to its success in fulfilling objectives and subobjectives.

Along with this establishment of the precedence of function over structure came another major decision, one involving fiscal responsibility: Every ASIM programmatic activity would not only be assigned according to objective, it would also have to conform to a budget whose funds were allocated by objective. The implication was clear: Henceforth, ASIM activities would have to survive a priority test; programs that made it within the budget allocation would be carried out, while lower priority items, no matter how strongly any one individual might advocate them, would not.

The familiar slogan that "the strength of ASIM lies with its component societies" received constant reinforcement. The *Component Society Officers Bulletin* continued to relay useful information to component leaders, keeping them up-to-date on what was going on nationally, and giving them strategies for upgrading their local function and for solving state-level problems—strategies that had often worked elsewhere. The Trustee assignment policy flourished. By the late seventies a Component Society Council was created at the national level, the sole function of which was to devise ways and means of helping component societies become more effective. A staff person was hired, Darryl Cardoza, who had as his principal assignment the health and welfare of components. Through a judicious blend of soft-sell and browbeating, he did his best to get laggard components to get their acts going. ASIM offered services to all components, some free, some on an at-cost basis. One service taken up sooner or later by all but the very largest components was the headquarters office's sophisticated capacity to bill for dues. Another was to publish newsletters. Good component societies, defined as those who increased their membership rolls, were given dues rebates. And, the very best societies were rewarded by getting an award at the Annual Meeting as Component Society of the Year, usually given for an array of problem-solving achievements.

But in reinforcing the work of components, ASIM did not forget its ultimate constituency, its rank-and-file members. In a variety of ways, ranging from the eminently practical to the purely educational, the Society looked after the interests of its members. It continued to offer them a variety of insurance programs for their use: in late 1972, adding a catastrophic liability policy and in early 1973, an excess major medical program. By 1973, the Insurance and Retirement Committee had arranged to make available to members the whole panoply of insurance plans—life insurance, disability, major medical, excess major medical, and a professional and personal liability umbrella. Along with insurance came an array of retirement plans—Keogh, profit-sharing, annuities, and two varieties of mutual funds. Incorporation, whether for group practice or solo practitioners, became a legal alternative for internists, and ASIM published dissertations in *The Internist* about the relative merits of incorporation or using the Keogh plan as a means of putting money away without tax liability.

In the early seventies, the Nixon Administration put wage and price controls into effect, at first for all segments of the economy and later for exclusive application to the presumably more inflationary health segment. Naturally, ASIM informed its members about the subtleties of the phase I-II-III regulations, even helping them decide how to raise their fees a little bit while still staying within the complex formula allowed by regulations.

A demographic survey of members was conducted in 1972 and subsequently published, revealing an array of useful facts. Three-quarters of the membership practiced general (as opposed to subspecialty) internal medicine; 93 percent had patient care as their principal activity (although more than half had another professional interest, principally teaching, with a sprinkling of others, such as administration, research, or industry); and the average age of members was 48.9 years (less than a year older than the 48.1 average a decade earlier; the 1977 figure, interestingly, was 51.7.)

The *Socioeconomic Handbook* went into its third edition, and, in 1972, headquarters announced that it had a socioeconomic bibliography available to those who wanted to research a subject for literary or practical use. Practice management workshops were conducted during the seventies, offering advice about billing, records, personnel practices, and other means of making an internist's practice more efficient.

The fact that a good many members had subspecialty interests, exclusive or part-time, was not forgotten. A series of subspecialty brochures ("Your Doctor Is a Cardiologist," "Your Doctor Is a Gastroenterologist," "Your Doctor Is an Allergist," etc.) was published in the early seventies, under the watchful editorial supervision of Ben Hall, their purpose being to explain to patients the scope and limits of subspecialty practice. For cardiology-minded internists, guidelines were published to help those reading electrocardiograms in hospitals to establish sound contractural agreements, and the virtues and flaws of computerized interpretation of EKGs were assessed and a summary disseminated.

Once it became clear that the College was going to get involved in socioeconomic matters, the Society's constraints against getting involved in educational matters were removed. In 1977, *The Internist* began publishing a regular monthly department, edited by New York's studious William Nelson (it was NYSSIM which had conceived the idea), called "Learning Goals: Curricula for Internists." Each month several pages of annotated bibliography were published, arranged by subspecialty, giving the key references in the recent literature for internist-readers to use in their continuing educational efforts.

For internists offering laboratory services in their offices, ASIM took the California SIM's lead. California had been one of the first states to require evidence of proficiency in the conduct of laboratory tests. In 1972, ASIM adapted a program developed by California SIM and offered the Medical Laboratory Evaluation (MLE) program. Through MLE, internists can obtain a certificate of competence in laboratory procedures if their lab's performance of "blind" lab tests measures up to standards.

Certain of ASIM's efforts for its members happily coincided with the Society's efforts in influencing national health policy. The long struggle to get third parties (including governmental health insurance agencies) to recognize Current Procedural Terminology (CPT) was matched by (and to some degree depended on the success of) ASIM's efforts to persuade all practicing internists to use the structured coding system in their billings to their patients.

Similarly, ASIM's long interest in improving medical records was channeled in the early seventies into the systematic problem-oriented method championed so evangelically by its inventor, Lawrence Weed. ASIM leapt quickly onto the problem-oriented medical record (POMR) bandwagon, modified the somewhat rigid original system for internists' everyday use, and promoted its adoption by internists in many ways, most notably through William Daines' eloquent handbook entitled "Handle For Care."

Of course, the more legible and orderly the medical record became, the more subject it was to being examined—and understood—by outsiders. This fact, combined with the increasingly litigious behavior of society and with the increasing use of electronic data processing to store, transmit and retrieve medical data, led to an increasing concern about possible damage to the confidential nature of the doctor/patient relationship. Characteristically, ASIM took prompt cognizance of this danger, appointed a task force, under Carmault Jackson, to study it, and by the mid-seventies had published a series of guidelines designed to help preserve the confidentiality of medical information, both for traditional and for computerized records.

In 1975, the malpractice crisis burst on the scene, and member internists began to have trouble securing malpractice insurance, while at the same time worrying about the increasing likelihood that they might be sued. Again, ASIM took prompt action. A task force, under Past President Glenn Molyneaux and later John Farrington, was appointed; it analyzed the situation, and published a paper describing the elements of the crisis and advising member internists how best to cope. ASIM considered forming a captive insurance company of its own for its members' use, but discarded the notion when it became clear that it was an exceedingly complex task and one of doubtful fiscal stability. Later in the seventies, Lonnie Bristow turned his seemingly limitless energies to the malpractice situation and successfully led a battle to get the Insurance Services Office (ISO) to soften its recommendations to malpractice insurers about classifying internists in regard to their performance of lumbar punctures, bone marrow aspirations, etc.

ASIM also felt a strong need to educate its members about matters which, although not then touching the day-to-day concerns of internists, had the potential of doing so. A good example is national health insurance, which during the seventies was constantly proclaimed as being "just around the corner." ASIM kept its members informed about developments through Annual Meeting programs, through the "Legislative Spotlight" column in *The Internist* (written at various times by William Felts, Thomas Gorsuch, Henry Blumberg, Thomas Connally and others), and through "comparative legislation" articles about Saskatchewan, England, Sweden, Denmark and other countries which had been through the experience.

Similarly, the Bennett amendment in 1973 changed peer review, long championed by ASIM as an honorable professional activity, from a purely private sector program to one funded by government. ASIM reacted in its now-familar pattern, appointing a task force, issuing white papers, working with the AMA, submitting testimony to a congressional committee in 1974, talking with other federal officials behind the scenes—and of course constantly informing the membership about it all. Health planning, drug regulation—including patient package inserts—Medicare amendments, and a host of other governmental incursions were reported faithfully to the members.

Nor did ASIM hesitate to discuss philosophical subjects with its members, matters that might have no direct impact on their practices or their pocketbooks but that might tease their intellect or influence their perceptions and attitudes. In 1973-74 a series of editorials (later bound together in a paperback book entitled *The Role of the Internist*) was published in consecutive issues of *The Internist,* their purpose being to lay out, in broad-brush strokes, where internists fit into the scheme of things.

The principal means of communication with rank-and-file members continued to be *The Internist.* As its circulation (mostly members, plus a sprinkling of health care "opinion-molders") increased from a few thousand in the sixties to more than 20,000 in 1980, it moved in small steps from a small, frankly amateur, inexpensively produced house organ to a smooth, polished professional-looking magazine. Some ASIM leaders wanted to call it a "journal," their argument being that its contents were designed for a professional audience and had some of the trappings of scientific papers; the majority held out for "magazine" on the grounds that the contents were designed less to give facts than to provoke thinking. In this context, the "magazine" model was not that of news or entertainment periodicals but of the intellectual monthlies.

While the content continued to be under the control and to reflect the interests of its practicing internist editor, the style and format of *The Internist* increasingly reflected the professional expertise and background of the staff assigned to it. At first there were staff editors, people like vivacious Laurie Spaulding, who had responsibility for all the chores of publication, including photography, typography, proofreading—and getting laggard authors to meet their deadlines. But later, as the scope of ASIM's communications efforts expanded, an overall Director of Communications position was created, filled by people with educational and experiential background in the field, first Bill Felch, Jr., later Connie Schantz, and now Barbara Lauter. Their cumulative efforts, along with a series of knowledgeable staff editors (Susan Anthony, Lynn Miller, and Diane Wigger among others) succeeded in changing *The Internist* from something a little bit stodgy to something a little bit slick.

By 1973, the familar old green masthead had disappeared, and the cover was now more often than not brightly colored, expertly designed and graphically evocative of the contents. Inside, there was now clean modern typography, with its ragged right columns, sidebars, lifted quotes and judicious use of color. In 1977, *The Internist* even published a supplement, this being a paperbound book on the proceedings of the memorable Conference on Ambulatory Care Review sponsored by ASIM in 1976, edited by Robert Hare. And in the late seventies, staff produced a series of practical, how-to inserts—bound into, but capable of being removed in toto from the middle of *The Internist*—dealing with such subjects as office personnel practices, use of computers, health insurance, and IPAs.

A change took place in the editorial content of *The Internist,* reflecting both the perceptions (biases?) of the successive editors—Furlong, Greene, Felch—and the changing scope of interests of the Society and its members. Some of the house organ features are still visible, such as "ASIM News" reporting which member was appointed to what important position. And another department, "ASIM Action," reports, as *The Internist* has always done, new Society policies, its positions on particular issues and the declarations it has made about them (often as testimony to various agencies of government).

It can be said that *The Internist* has gone through three stages in its editorial content. First, it was a house organ, occupied with *describing* ASIM activities and the leaders who accomplished them. Second, while continuing to report ASIM's affairs, it now began to *interpret* their significance, placing them in the context of the entire health care arena. Third, it is now no longer beholden to current ASIM activities to decide what it will publish; today, the editor and his staff are *selective* about their topics, choosing months ahead of time what theme will be presented in each issue, picking prominent authors to argue that theme from several viewpoints, highlighting it with an editorial or an overview. Sometimes, miniature membership surveys are included, or bits of humor are added; occasionally, a subtheme is explored. The result has been that over the past several years, *The Internist* has presented explications of nearly all of the major health care issues. In some instances, for example catastrophe health insurance, the magazine has been ahead of the game, discussing complex aspects of a topic before they had been generally debated in public policy forums. In any event, an ASIM member who keeps his *Internist* accessible on the library shelf will sooner or later have on tap a reference library of the significant issues in today's health care field.

3

The Move to Washington

Advantageous Address

A convincing argument can be made that ASIM was the first medical specialty society to recognize the importance of governmental incursions into the health care arena. From the beginning, the Society had had a legislative committee, and over the years, its leaders reacted to various legislative or regulatory initiatives by submitting testimony to congressional committees, to governmental agencies, or—in one-to-one conversations—to representatives from the White House or Capitol Hill.

The major social legislation of the mid-sixties convinced the ASIM leadership about two significant points. First, the Society had demonstrated its capacity—through a major, bootstrap, ad hoc effort—to deal effectively with important legislation, both in influencing its course and in educating members about its impact on them and their patients. Second, while this improvisational approach was demonstrably successful, probably because of the formidable intellectual and organizational powers that internist-leaders seemed to possess, it was still not as effective as a different strategy might be. What was needed was more sustained exposure to the legislative process, more regular contact with the people making it go (sometimes legislative staffers even more than their bosses), and more frequent opportunity, formal and informal, to make ASIM positions heard. Using these tactics was nearly impossible for an organization whose headquarters office was 3,000 miles away from the Potomac.

James Feffer, during his presidency in 1967-68, took cognizance of the situation and, characteristically refusing to accept the status quo as immutable, appointed a committee under William Felch to study the possibility of moving the Society away from its San Francisco home. The committee found many things in favor of moving eastward. Liaison with other professional organizations, for instance, would be facilitated—particularly if the move were to Chicago. Staff travel expense to meetings would lessen. Most persuasive, a move to Washington would be a move to the place where the action is. But the committee, when it looked at one major piece of information, didn't waste much time in deciding on a negative recommendation to the Board. The cost of a move would be prohibitive, consuming more than the Society had in its reserve fund at the time. The idea was dropped. The San Francisco sentimentalists breathed easier; those afflicted with Potomac fever took some aspirin and waited.

The benefits of doing things at the Washington locus were not lost sight of. In May 1975, when ASIM happened to have its Annual Meeting in the nation's capital, a new strategy was introduced, called the "Congressional Visits Project." (Staff, of course, called it CVP, unaware that internists generally reserve those initials to mean "central venous pressure.") The notion had been conceived by ASIM's Liaison Council, the campaign had been planned by staff, and the appointments had been made by individual component members. The result: Nearly all of the state component society delegations attending the Annual Meeting had one or more of their members assigned to talk to a Senator or Representative from "back home." Cadres of ASIM internists had separate meetings with the chairmen of the four major congressional committees dealing with health—Senators Edward Kennedy and Russell Long, Congressmen Paul Rogers and Al Ullman. The conversations lasted from a few minutes to more than an hour, and discussions mostly revolved around health legislation (although one senator took time to arrange a physical exam appointment for his wife). Sometimes administrative assistants substituted for a legislator, but the visiting internists' disappointment usually evaporated when they found the staff aide to be knowledgeable and sophisticated about health matters. When the CVP was over, and the internist-visitors had been debriefed and their impressions and reactions collated, there was general agreement that the project had been successful and was worth repeating. It was done again in October 1977, with even more impressive results. Henceforth, it was agreed, when ASIM wanted its positions disseminated to influential legislators, it could be done with the likelihood that the personal contact from constituent internists would be remembered.

Some ten years after the initial discussion of a move in 1968, the idea surfaced again. This time it was Bill Ramsey and his staff, working with the Board's Executive Committee, who explored the pros and cons of a move. The target this time was obviously Washington. The principal argument was much the same: key staff and key elected leaders spent much of their time up in the air (literally speaking; in the figurative sense, their feet were always on the ground) traveling to or from the D.C. seat of power. The chief negative argument no longer applied: The Society could now afford a cross-country move, through the use of roughly a third of the reserve fund that had been so carefully built up over the years for emergency needs of the Society. Most key staff members would be willing to pull up their roots (although, inevitably, a couple of useful ones had their hearts so completely committed to San Francisco that even an enticing bonus could not lure them East). The principal negative argument now was simply that the Society might get too deeply embroiled in the political scene.

When the topic of the move was presented to the House of Delegates in May 1978 (the Bylaws gave the Board the right to make the decision, but the Trustees thought it wise to get the House's endorsement), the discussion didn't last too long. To be sure, there was a past president or two recalling the Society's long-term roots in San Francisco, their comments receiving a sentimental round of applause. And a persistent argument came from worriers expressing fears that ASIM might succumb to Potomac fever and concentrate only on political activities to the detriment of its other concerns.

But the Board and staff had done their homework too well. Every argument (including the alternative of having a Washington branch office 3,000 miles away from headquarters) was countered successfully. In the end, it seemed that most everybody favored the move as being in ASIM's best interests, and agreed that the resistance was largely perfunctory and "for the record." At the final House session, the reference committee recommendation for endorsing the move was passed unanimously.

Once the decision was approved by all parties, Bill Ramsey's staff set to work to accomplish the myriad tasks involved in the logistics of the move—securing new office space in the D.C. area, assisting staff members who would move and replacing those who would not, translocating furniture and equipment, touching necessary legal bases, and many others. Staff worked overtime during the rest of 1978. Late that year, a little more than six months after the die had been cast, the move was made. A couple of months after moving into its new, permanent quarters, ASIM announced its arrival to official Washington with a cocktail reception attended by Congressmen, agency representatives, and the ASIM leadership.

By the summer of 1981, ASIM was 25 years old and had been headquartered for a tenth of that time in Washington, D.C. Barring a few wistful backward glances by an occasional staff member still hungering for San Francisco, no regrets are voiced. Everyone—ASIM leaders, its staff, its components, its members—seems to agree that the brave decision to move was also a good one. ASIM has settled comfortably into the Washington scene. Its presence is felt there, both through its regular staff members (Bill Ramsey and his aides) and more recently the staff lobbyist, Richard Trachtman. ASIM leaders find it comparatively simple to fly in, conduct some piece of business with the executive or the legislative branch of government, and fly home again.

Worries about Potomac fever have proven groundless. Staff members, to be sure, are partly caught up in the excitement of the daily intricacies of politics. But their sense of balance—their commitment to the full range of goals and objectives that are on the ASIM agenda—prevails. Washington has turned out to be a good place for ASIM to be, not just for its political interests, but also for its traditional social and economic ones.

4

ASIM Leaders

Acclaim for Attainment

As was true during its first 15 years, ASIM has serendipitously managed in the last ten years to produce a plethora of effective leaders, individuals who somehow provided the right set of skills at the right time. Witness its elected leaders.

In 1971, ASIM's president was Otto Page, a soft-spoken but articulate internist from Portland, Oregon, champion of the efficient practice of internal medicine both through good medical records and the effective use of allied health professionals. Expert in the mechanics of practice, he was equally at home in dealing with legislators and with the amalgamation excitement.

The following year, Edwin Evans rose to the top job. Cool, unflappable and unmoved by time pressures (a possibly apocryphal story has it that the sometimes compulsive Bill Ramsey saw fit to take off his wristwatch during this presidential year), this Atlanta internist was equally comfortable welcoming Julie Nixon Eisenhower to a breakfast meeting at that year's Las Vegas Interim Meeting and offering testimony against flawed legislative proposals.

In 1973, William Campbell Felch took over the presidential reins. This Rye, New York group practitioner, ready with the spoken and the written word, tried to fulfill his promise that ASIM would be willing to meet "with anyone, anytime, anywhere" by traveling to Chicago, to Washington and to more than half the Society's components, while somehow finding the time to write monthly columns about the "Role of the Internist."

In 1974, ASIM, turning once again to its San Francisco roots, elected energetic Glenn Molyneaux as its chief officer. Tireless (he insisted upon flying "red-eye" night flights to and from California so as to fulfill the dual demands of practice and of Society work), he managed to combine his enthusiasm for furthering ASIM's economic and operational efficiency with his interest in special issues, such as primary care, health insurance, and malpractice.

Ralph Reinfrank, chief of medicine at the Hartford Hospital, was the next to bring his special talents to ASIM's top position. Wry, and dedicated to erasing "Mickey Mouse" methods from ASIM operations, he brought a rare level of intellectual sophistication to the spoken and written word and a consummate ability to cut through chaff to get to the wheat.

In 1976, the new president was William R. Felts. Long ASIM's "man in Washington," the fact that he had friends in high places and a consuming interest in legislative and regulatory affairs did not mean that he did not also have the capacity to work toward improving internists' comprehension of other subjects, including CPT, the use of computers, and the pitfalls of socialized health systems elsewhere in the world.

The next president, Ogden, Utah internist William P. Daines, although quiet and non-assertive by nature, has left a strong mark on ASIM in a host of ways. Whether it is the procedural rules for reference committees, the problem-oriented medical record, the recertification process, the flaws of the CME enterprise, modern management methods for ASIM operations, or the design of the budget, the fine hand of "Purdie" Daines can be found in all.

In 1978, Ben Hall combined his homespun eastern Tennessee style with some innate personal political sagacity and brought them to bear on the big job. Equally at home with the conceptual aspects of quality assurance and the practical requirements of brochure writing, he was a principal figure in the early development of FCIM, and was ASIM's president during its momentous transcontinental headquarters move.

In 1979, James Collins became ASIM's second president from Pennsylvania. Chief of the Geisinger Clinic in Danville, previously known as the Board's quiet man, he showed as its chairman a remarkable capacity for keeping ASIM affairs on track—and keeping his sometimes unruly colleagues from wandering afield. He led the Society in a period of external strain with the College and in a time of internal strengthening of component societies.

ASIM's 24th president, Colorado's John Farrington, will have served more months in that capacity than any of his predecessors, the shift of the Annual Meeting from spring to fall having created for him a sixteen-month-plus term of office. A steady and indefatigable toiler, he has (up to this writing) presided over a time in which ASIM has consolidated its national credibility while at the same time making necessary adjustments to sweeping changes imposed by a new administration in Washington.

On the Society's 25th birthday, it will figuratively return to its California roots when the San Francisco Bay Area's Lonnie Bristow ascends to the top job. Obviously, no one can predict what pressures, strains, or crises will face the Society during his regime. But ASIM members can feel confident that their 25th president, like all his predecessors, will bring to the task a rich mixture of talents and skills sufficient to meet all challenges.

These eleven leaders and their fourteen predecessors are now (or will be when their tours are completed) members of the exclusive George Wever Club, the only qualification for membership being that one is a past ASIM president. Working for ASIM must breed vitality and longevity: only two of its past presidents have died, the second, Bert Persons, and the fifth, Ross Taylor.

In the 1970s, as before, a number of internists made valuable contributions to ASIM as Trustees, yet, for one reason or another, did not become president. Blaine Hibbard finished his long tour of service, finally as secretary-treasurer, in 1972. Frank Riddick resigned in 1975 after seven years on the Board, to devote full time to his position as director of New Orleans' Ochsner Clinic, although he stayed on as ASIM's delegate to the AMA House until 1980. Ohio's William Millhon served eight years on the Board, notably involved in the ASPERF project (for which he mounted a pilot test in Columbus) and as an ASIM representative to the ABIM Board. Wisconsin's Mike Mehr and Florida's John Verner served short but useful terms on the Board before other, more pressing, demands on their time forced them to resign. Mervin Shalowitz served the Board with distinction through nearly the whole of the seventies, his special forte being ASIM's internal affairs (membership, finances, insurance, etc.) and his championing of a group practice, fee-for-service variety of HMO. Texas' Carmault Jackson served for three years, his special field of expertise being computerized systems and the need for protecting confidentiality within them.

There are other good and useful citizens of ASIM on the Board in 1981, and only a crystal ball could detect for sure which of them will end up being members of the George Wever Club—except for New York's Monte Malach whose nomination as president-elect will be voted on at the October 1981 annual session. Other old hand members of the Board are John Abrums, Albuquerque's bow-tied expert on parliamentary behavior, health insurance and solo practice, and Reggie Harris, North Carolina's ebullient champion of primary care and management systems. Next come N. Thomas Connally, ASIM's latest "man in Washington" and thoughtful interpreter of both legislative and non-legislative national perspectives, Burns Roehrig, Massachusetts' learned connoisseur of components and cognitive services, and Warren Tingley, Texas' articulate proponent of rationality.

Then there is another duo, Oregon's Robert Hare, persuasive advocate of performance assessment, and Ohio's Paul Metzger, who effortlessly can look at health insurance both from the consumer (practicing internist) and the provider (company exec) viewpoint. And the newest pair on the Board are New Jersey's Emanuel Abraham, highly organized proponent of peer review, and Michigan's Joseph Sentkeresty, solid advocate of influencing organized medicine.

Assisting the Board in accomplishing its work are a series of committees and task forces, some of which are chaired by non-trustees: Health Systems Agencies Committee—New York's Sidney Weinstein; Ambulatory Systems Task Force—Virginia's James Nuckolls; Health Insurance Benefits Committee—Washington, D.C.'s Charles Duvall; Institutional Relationships Committee—Oregon's Donald Olson; Medical Liability Committee—California's George Bauer; Pharmaceuticals and Therapeutics Committee—Baltimore's Thaddeus Prout; Task Force on Cost-Effectiveness—Illinois' Hugh Espey; Geriatrics—Tennessee's Lyman Fulton; Unions—New York's Norman Blackman; Bylaws—Pennsylvania's Ray Grandon; Insurance and Retirement—Texas' R. Andrew Jackson; Investment—Pennsylvania's Robert Pressman; Laboratories—Illinois' Donald Hanscom (Trustee designee up for a vote at the October meeting); Manpower and Primary Care—New York's William Dermody; and Meetings—Oregon's Spence Meighan.

What happens to old ASIM hands after their tour of duty? The most common pattern, of course—and this has been true throughout the quarter century—is to retreat from center stage and return to the pre-limelight existence, usually in the private practice of internal medicine. But ASIM leaders seem to have some intrinsic capacity for leadership, and it is not at all uncommon for the headquarters office to get word that Dr. A was made chief of staff at his hospital, that Dr. B was elected president of the county medical society, and that Dr. C now presides over the state heart association. It is noteworthy that not a few one-time ASIM leaders (at component or national level) subsequently became Governors of the ACP and a couple reached high office in the College (Marvin Pollard, an early ASIM trustee, became ACP president; Max Berry, an ASIM president, and Carter Smith, a Society Trustee, were later College Regents).

The Internist has a regular feature, "ASIM News," which reports the ascension of ASIM members to high office in the ranks of organized medicine. This is done evenhandedly, the announcement being the same in size and tone whether the individual in question is a rank-and-file member or a past president.

In recent years, quite a group of ASIM members have become presidents of state medical associations: New Mexico—John Abrums, District of Columbia—Ray Scalletar, Pennsylvania—Ray Grandon, Georgia—Charlie Hollis, North Carolina—William Kelly, California—Joseph Boyle.

The AMA's governing structure is laced with not a few past or current ASIM members, either grassroots or leadership: Legislation—Morse Kochtitzky, Clinton McGill, William Felch, William Golden; Medical Services—Lonnie Bristow, John Finkbeiner, Raymond Scalettar; Medical Education—Patrick Corcoran, George Thoma, Jr., Frank Riddick; Long Range Planning—Joseph Painter; Scientific Affairs—C. John Tupper, Ira Friedlander; AMA Education and Research Foundation—George Mills, Alan Nelson. The AMA Board's two top positions, chairman and vice chairman, were held by ASIM members up until June 1981: Lowell Steen of Indiana and Joseph Boyle of California (who succeeded Steen as chairman at that time). Other members of the Board are Utah's Alan Nelson and Hawaii's George Mills. AMA's House of Delegates, which seats slightly more than 250 persons, has numbered among them, on the average over the last decade, some 40 to 50 members of ASIM.

The National Academy of Science was chartered in 1863 by President Lincoln to provide the federal government with expert policy advice on scientific matters, but it was not until 1970 that a separate division was chartered, called the Institute of Medicine (IOM) and charged with generating expert policy positions on important health issues. The total elected membership of the prestigious IOM in 1980 was 378 (out of a charter-stipulated maximum of 400), of whom slightly more than 10 percent come from the ranks of private practitioners. The list as a whole includes a sizable number of ASIM members. There are six ASIM presidents (Bristow, Daines, Evans, Felch, Felts, Watts), three former Trustees (Jackson, Riddick, Richard Wilbur), three past recipients of ASIM's Distinguished Internist of the Year award (Harvey Estes, Saul Farber, Dwight Wilbur), a group who have seen active service on ASIM councils, committees or components (Langdon Burwell, William Dowda, Fred Gilbert, the late Michael Halberstam, Alan Nelson, Alvin Thompson), and a cluster of others who, though coming with other credentials, have had occasion to work closely with the ASIM leadership in a variety of forums (among others, ACP leaders Stuart Bondurant, John Gamble, James Haviland, Robert Petersdorf).

Some ASIM luminaries gravitate into the groves of academe, as did James Feffer and Malcolm Watts. Others, like Joseph Painter and Frank Riddick, lend their skills to managing large medical institutions. Still others, including Robert Long and Paul Metzger, hold high posts in the health insurance industry. ASIM members have been involved with industry (IBM, Control Data Corporation, the Bell System), with government (the PSRO Board), with politics (Reagan/Bush advisory groups), with economics (National Commission on the Cost of Medical Care), with hospitals (the AHA Committee on Physicians), and with continuing medical education (the Alliance For Continuing Medical Education and the new AACME).

Indeed, in 1981 it is difficult to think of a major health care arena that does not have at least one ASIM member involved in its activities. And it is a safe assumption that these internists, whatever their current milieu is, will bring with them some habits acquired during their ASIM years—the cool, thoughtful, analytical, reasoned approach that characterizes the ASIM method.

5

ASIM/SEREF
Accent on Advocacy

Smaller siblings are frequently beset with identity problems because of uncertain relationships with older and stronger big brothers. So it was with ASIM's kid sibling, the Socio-Economic Research and Education Foundation (SEREF).

Serif's mission was clear enough—to foster projects designed to put the delivery of medical care on a sound scientific basis. The problem lay in deciding how to go about achieving that end. It was not that there was a dearth of identifiable projects that would be worthy of ASIM's support. Right from the Society's first years, its leaders sought better, more valid ways to identify internists' services precisely; SEREF's first project was a joint exploration with the University of Michigan of a method to accomplish that task, and several years of effort were spent—in vain, it turned out—in designing a suitable technique. Over the years, many other schemes have presented themselves, involving the array of internists' interests—coding and nomenclature, record-keeping, use of technology, process of care analysis, auditing, cost containment, health education, and others—and most such offerings were deemed to be worthy of pursuit.

Certainly, the vehicle to do the job was there. SEREF, as a 501-C-3 not-for-profit corporation, was entitled to receive money from donors who could deduct such gifts for tax purposes. And there was an abundance of talent within the Society to evaluate project applications for rigor of design and worthwhileness of intent.

The difficulty, of course, lay with resources, specifically the lack of same. Unlike other foundations whose very names—Kellogg, Rockefeller, Ford, Robert Wood Johnson—conjure up images of wealth, SEREF has always been dependent on current donations, principally from ASIM internists. Members are offered the opportunity, with their annual Society dues renewal, to make a contribution to SEREF, and an astonishing number do so, winning a tax deduction and the right to wear the blue SEREF button on their name tags at ASIM meetings. It should not be thought that member solicitation always produces trivial sums; in 1974, when the Society was dedicated to implementing its ASPERF project, it took the unusual step of mounting a campaign to get internists, members and later non-members, to contribute $100. The result was an astonishing $100,000, an amount sufficient to permit the pilot phase of ASPERF to proceed.

SEREF does not depend exclusively on member donations. Big brother ASIM, with its more dependable revenue sources, has made a practice of donating annual lump sums to its frailer sibling; most years, it has awarded $10,000, chiefly for SEREF to accomplish its basic administrative chores.

For a while in the sixties and early seventies, SEREF's energetic president, Florida's Robert Raborn, dreamed of getting private individuals and businesses to make what fund raisers call "significant" contributions to SEREF. He organized a group of friends and patients (called by some scoffers the Del Ray Mafia) and succeeded for a while in getting a modest influx of dollars into SEREF coffers.

But the fact is that, with rare exceptions, SEREF has not had sufficient revenues to be able, by itself, to fund major projects. It has, of course, served as a channel for other funding sources, the best example being the 1970 HEW-funded study of the office care of internists conducted by ASIM under Oregon's Robert Hare and ASIM staff member Shlomo Barnoon. At other times, it has been a partner in funding with others, contributing money for one segment of a worthy project (for example, the current project on cognitive services).

One question has troubled SEREF Boards over the years: To what degree should SEREF be passive, waiting for worthy projects to show up for consideration, and to what degree should the Foundation be active, conceiving and designing and conducting its own projects? The answer has varied from time to time, but most Boards have thought both strategies should be employed, depending on current situations and the current size of the bank account.

This ongoing debate about function also inevitably stirs up a companion argument about structure, especially concerning the interrelationship between the siblings. In the beginning, the linkages were close: members of the ASIM Board were automatically members of the SEREF Board, and decisions about one organization could easily take into account the needs of the other. Later, it was deemed helpful to give SEREF some autonomy, with separate officers (except for secretary-treasurer, a position which has always had the ASIM officer also serving the SEREF Board), and with some SEREF Board members not serving on the Society Board (although for a while the slots were occupied in part by Society past presidents). At one point, there was feeling that SEREF was too much a creature of ASIM and that it should strive to further the broader interests of society instead of just the narrow concerns of internists. An advisory board was appointed which met and prepared positions about societal health needs (health education was a prominent one). The effort was sincere and the product reasonable; unhappily, it promptly ran into the familiar barrier: no funds for implementation.

Interlocking or independent, all SEREF Boards have faced one more question: What mechanism should be used in evaluating various notions, concepts, project ideas or detailed programs that come knocking on the SEREF door? In particular, what objective analysis can SEREF employ to screen potential projects, including those pet ideas submitted by loyal—and perhaps eminent—ASIM members? Ralph Reinfrank was responsible for devising the mechanism which is still used—a quality evaluation committee, beholden to no one, responsible only for rigorous analysis of projects. Yet the committee has the power to approve, disapprove or return for clarification or modification; its decisions are strictly on the merits of the project—its research design and feasibility of implementation—and not on its funding or strategic ramifications, which are left to other bodies.

By its very nature, a fundless foundation is no fun. In such a situation, identity problems are not only possible, they are likely. These were so intrinsic and fundamental that they could not be promptly resolved by ASIM's standard problem-solving techniques. Over the years, a number of tasks forces and ad hoc committees wrestled with the question of what to do about SEREF and failed to come up with a facile answer.

Failing the usual brainpower solution, ASIM has had to settle for empiricism. Various structural approaches have been deployed and various functional models tested. Fortunately, the Society was once again blessed with a series of topnotch individuals to explore alternative routes. Robert Raborn brought an entrepreneurial, marketing talent to the task, one that was foreign to conservative Trustees but horizon-expanding for others. Cleveland's Ed Hahn pushed the pendulum back a ways, bringing a more traditional, organized-medicine style to SEREF activities. Buffalo's Robert Kohn had a vision of an expanded role for the Foundation, but was frustrated by skeptical traditionalists on big brother's Board. Finally, William Smith has brought his Oklahoma quiet and thorough steadiness to the top slot.

Today, more than two decades after its creation, SEREF seems to have found its legitimate place in the ASIM family. The trials and tribulations of growing up have rubbed off the rough edges. SEREF will never be a huge Robert Wood Johnson kind of foundation. But neither will it vanish from the scene, starved to death by lack of greenback nourishment. SEREF has found its modest niche in the facilitation of a limited number of worthy projects, things it can afford to support and to assist in achieving worthy outcomes. Its relationships with big brother have finally been worked out, to their mutual satisfaction.

Like other parts of the ASIM family, the Foundation sibling has grown up to become a mature adult.

6

ASIM Staff

Accomplished Agents

A mark of organizational maturity is the degree to which relationships have been worked out between the voluntary leadership and the paid staff. Ordinarily, the separation of powers is clearly defined in charters or bylaws, with the former having ultimate authority and responsibility for organizational affairs, for establishment of policy, for reviewing the past, for evaluating the present and planning for the future, and for the assignment of the execution of policy. The latter is the principal executor of policy, carries out defined tasks and responsibilities, administers internal functions, and assesses operational effectiveness.

Sharp as these paper distinctions seem, they frequently blur and overlap in the real world to such a degree that, for quite a few organizations, the mix is troubling and even disruptive. For one thing, voluntary leaders (delegates, officers, trustees, committee members) are nearly always part-time toilers in the field; they have other interests, including the critical one of making a living; only a portion of their energies is committed to organizational goals. Staff members, by definition, are full-time; their commitment to the organization is high since their livelihood comes from it. A frequent result of such differences is an impatience on the part of dedicated staff with a perceived lack of commitment from titular leaders.

Another internecine problem arises from the fact that voluntary leaders are transient, appearing on the scene, having their day of glory, then disappearing, while staff members are permanent (to the degree that they are competent and for as long as the organization can satisfy their career aspirations). The result often is that staff members see themselves as having more sophistication than their employers, particularly neophyte ones, who are perceived as regularly reinventing the wheel.

These dilemmas can create trouble in organizations and can lead at times to opposite—and equally harmful—solutions: too strong a staff or too weak a staff.

ASIM managed to escape these traps. The separation of powers has always been clearly understood by both parties, and problems relating to role and function have simply not arisen. Partly, this happy state of affairs has come about because of the nature of ASIM's voluntary leaders—their willingness, even compulsion, during the time they are in charge, to assume the mantle of leadership and to make the necessary commitment of time and energy to fulfill the leadership role.

Perhaps to a greater degree, ASIM's successful delineation of the complementary roles has been brought about by the fact that its role-conscious executive, Bill Ramsey, has insisted on it. At one level, he has demanded that timorous or doubtful Trustees make up their minds among alternative courses of action; a favorite phrase is "You guys decide." Simultaneously, he is scrupulous (and insists that his staff members observe a similar scrupulosity) about not inching over a finely drawn line. He and his staff will always provide information about a subject. They will usually display the array of possible solutions. They will, if asked, list the pros and cons of a particular course. They can proffer the collective staff recommendation—but only when the subject relates to fiscal, legal or administrative topics falling within staff's jurisdiction. But they will never volunteer an opinion on a major Society policy or strategy matter; if pressed for such an opinion, they will likely hedge or, reluctantly, indicate a mild preference.

The caliber of ASIM staff members has been such that it must not have been easy for them to observe the fine line of separation. Dorothy Titland, who came on board as a secretary in 1963, has become the Society's Board secretary, in which capacity she has had to listen to repeated discussions about the same topics. Her forbearance in getting it all down is remarkable; her only complaint about Board meetings, one senses, is that the male Board members may be physiologically tuned to a different periodicity than hers. The quality of her work is shown by the excellence of her minutes, and by the way in which, wearing another chapeau, she manages to understand ASIM's insurance and retirement program offerings as well as those committee chairmen in charge of it, the perennial Harmon Harvey and now, for two years, the ebullient Andrew Jackson.

Another long-time staffer was David Kahn, who has now moved on to a top dog position elsewhere. Associate Director (back when the staff was much smaller), Kahn's deliberate, sometimes plodding work style stood in sharp contrast to his twinkle-toed tap dancing and other terpsichorean talents.

Mark Leasure came from Ohio to San Francisco and finally to Washington, gradually turning into staff's political pundit, hiding—under a homespun country boy exterior—a sharp mind, an articulate speaking ability (he was a featured speaker at ASIM's 1979 Annual Meeting), and a ready wit. His sidekick, Darryl Cardoza, used his distinctive blend of toughness and charm to whip laggard component societies into shape. Both of these outstanding staff members chose ASIM's 25th year to move on to other careers. Still on board, and newest staff legislative expert, is Bob Doherty, whose youthful mien is contradicted by his deep voice and the mature way he uses it.

In the communications department, there first was Bill Felch, Jr., whose worrying intelligence was able to encompass both the entire forest and twigs on individual trees—and who, though a transplanted Easterner, refused to leave San Francisco for Washington. In Washington, the position was taken over by Connie Schantz, talented writer, idea promoter, and competent administrator. She melded all three of these skills in her staff assignment to get this history out on time—and is only leaving for the more important job of raising a family. And now there is Barbara Lauter whose vitality and vivacity are astonishing, and who knows her way around the communications byways.

Wendy Smith, simultaneously quiet and forceful, staffs an eclectic mix of committees and task forces. Her summaries are such a model of clarity and interpretation that her committee chairmen are allowed to ignore the unwritten rule that chairmen should write their own minutes and to delegate that task to her superior talent.

A host of other staff have come, left their mark, and moved on—Ed Daleske, Steve Passin, Nadia Plyer, Sandi Dutra, Bill Burke, Stephanie Dimitroff, to name a few.

A few others, who shall remain nameless, have come, been unable to keep up with ASIM's performance standards—measured by process (long hours of work) and outcomes (the impossible getting done)—and have shortly departed from the scene.

And it should not be forgotten that the names listed above have been those of top staff persons. Working with them have been a host of secretaries, clerks, programmers, editorial assistants, printers, accountants, etc.—all the variety of people needed to make a large and complex operation work—and work well.

And, in charge of all 31 of them, at the top of the staff pyramid for nearly 15 years now, is the redoubtable William R. Ramsey, who has presided over the expansion of the ASIM operation from a small, somewhat homey, almost amateur, one into today's large, smoothly oiled, professionally run machine. And this has been accomplished carefully, in small increments, with Board leaders understanding and approving each step. And it has been done without losing the personal touch: he is still accessible not only to ASIM big guns but also to any grassroots member. A telephone caller, seeking some information to be found or some chore to be done, can hang up, knowing it will be accomplished.

Like every top dog, he has had stones cast at him. Some say he has favorites, both among staff and Trustees; of course he does, but he's remarkably evenhanded. Some say he has mood swings; normally equable, his anxiety titer naturally escalates before Board meetings and especially before Annual Meetings. One past president accused him—jokingly—of being paranoid; he's not, he's just normally suspicious of anyone not a dyed-in-the-wool ASIM supporter. He disparages the political games played at AMA meetings, but he also revels in them. "Don't just talk to each other," he urges ASIM Executive Committee members, "Get out there and *be visible*." He loves California and looks forward to a more peaceful existence there sometime in the future; but he enjoys the Washington scene too, and is sure that ASIM was right in moving to "where the action is. . . ."

The proof, of course, is in the pudding—or, put in ASIM lingo—outcomes are the best measure of performance. Bill Ramsey's staff has been remarkably loyal to him; it is said that the give-and-take at the staff meetings held to discuss ways and means of advancing ASIM are open, spirited, sometimes argumentative, but nearly always end in development of consensus.

How does the voluntary leadership assess this man? The answer is clear: the Board in 1978 took the unusual step (nearly unheard of for a non-MD exec of an organization whose members are all physicians) of giving Bill Ramsey the title of executive vice president. The action signifies confidence, affection, and—especially—trust.

7

Learning at Meetings
Artistic Annuals

Of the many examples of ways in which the ASIM of the seventies addressed its problems in a grown-up way, a particularly good one is found in the manner in which it planned and mounted its Annual Meetings.

For years, these displays of the Society's sophistication had been put on in what might be called "the old way." A single Trustee, usually chosen because the meeting was being held in or near his home town, would be in charge. He would be responsible, perhaps with a small committee to help, for planning everything, not only the programmatic content but also the social events, spouses' activities, entertainment, and logistics.

It should not be thought that these one-man shows necessarily turned out a flawed product. The quintessential instance of a successful production was the 1968 meeting in Frank Foster's Boston. While perfect baked beans and pluperfect scrod may not have been in evidence, there were nonetheless other tokens of the Athens of the U.S., including a lengthy lecture by the editor-in-chief of the *Christian Science Monitor,* Edwin Canham, and an elegant reception at the majestic Boston Museum of Fine Arts.

The 1972 meeting in Atlantic City, perhaps because there was no Trustee from New Jersey, was more eclectic than elegant. Wilbur Mills, then still the all-powerful chairman of the House Ways and Means Committee, spoke to a packed house at the luncheon meeting, endearing himself to ASIM attendees by calling Trustee William R. Felts "Billy Bob." The banquet speaker was octogenarian Paul Dudley White, renowed cardiologist, who described his view of "Medicine in the People's Republic of China" in such detail that he nearly missed his plane.

In 1973, the site was Chicago. As usual, the aim was to get "big names" for the program, and, as usual, the aim was realized. FDA Commissioner Charles Edwards was there to talk about regulation. So was Senator Wallace Bennett, optimistic author of the PSRO legislation. The luncheon speaker was John Hogness, the president of the Institute of Medicine.

But successful though these sessions were, it was becoming increasingly evident that planning national meetings for ASIM was no one-man job. For one thing, the Society was now putting on two program sessions a year, a fall Interim Meeting in addition to the spring Annual Meeting. At first, the Interim Meetings were small carbon copies of the annual events, aiming for big topics and big names (and held in distinctive locations like Dallas, Cambridge, and Portland). But it soon became apparent that this was too much of a good thing. The Interim sessions, it was decided, should focus on the component societies and should deal with practical matters (i.e. communications, problem-oriented records, negotiating techniques, the liability crisis), often using how-to workshops. The Annual Meeting would continue to lay stress on the big issues (PSRO, health planning, national health insurance, primary care, manpower, hospitals, recertification, etc.) and would bring in the big guns to discuss them.

The complex task of organizing these meetings could not be handled on an ad hoc, one-year-at-a-time, basis. Planning and continuity of effort was needed. To be sure, Bill Ramsey's increasingly competent staff could take over the logistical effort, the infinite number of mechanical details relating to such mundane matters as meals, microphones, and media. But the program content surely required the internist's viewpoint, and the logical solution was to appoint a Meetings Committee to decide what should be presented and who should present it. At first, a Board member was chosen to oversee this important function. But it soon became apparent that among the ASIM membership are a few who have a natural bent for this kind of thing, and first the ingenious Alan Nelson and now the inimitable Scot, Spence Meighan, have risen to chair the Committee.

The changes wrought by these incessantly inventive chairmen—aided in no small part by some talented and tough committee members (Jerry Applebaum, Michael Perry, David Taylor, among others)—indicate once again the self-confidence that maturity begets. The new programmatic style makes use of breezy alliteration: the 1977 Annual Meeting was entitled "Battle for the Buck." It can make small jokes: in 1979, the Annual Meeting (held in New Orleans) was called "Medicine—and All That Jazz;" and the Interim Meeting (held in Las Vegas) bore the title "What's in the Cards?"

The aim today is to stimulate, even provoke, the audience, and the level of provocation depends on the manner of the presentation. Formal debates serve the purpose well; so do playlets, slide shows and participatory workshops. Content can still focus on the big issues (the 1978 Annual Meeting—entitled "Medical Care, Ltd."—included discussions of PSROs, HMOs, health planning, drug reform, and rationing of medical care), but balance is achieved by interspersing some touches of closer-to-home material (in 1976, a psychiatrist's somewhat critical analysis of the typical internist's personality traits evoked a spate of somewhat defensive letters to the editor). Big names are still sought, but only if those bearing them are also stimulating speakers (the two, one observes, do not always go hand-in-hand); lesser lights are at times preferable, especially if two or more of them can be persuaded to engage in frank exchanges of differences of opinion. To keep the pot boiling, members of the Committee are drafted to chair the various segments of the program; often called moderator, their real role is to stir up immoderate interchanges.

These innovations, permitted at first somewhat grudgingly by tradition-bound Trustees, are now accepted by Board and rank-and-file members alike, as the epitome of modern, multi-media professional programming. The post-meeting evaluation sheets circulated by the Continuing Physician Education Advisory Committee (SEREF's vehicle for gaining accreditation so as to permit the awarding of Category 1 credit) nearly always give highly favorable marks to the program sessions. Reporters from *The Internist* write up the proceedings in some detail, their instructions being to capture the flavor as well as the substance of what went on. All sessions are now recorded professionally, and a modest market has been found willing to purchase the tapes for later study and reflection.

Clyde Greene's wrap-up speech to the House as his presidential term ended (for some years, *The Internist* called such dissertations the "exaugural" address until some pedant looked it up and found that no such word exists) was entitled "We've Come a Long Way Maybe." This phrase captures (understandably, if not elegantly) the essence of the changes in ASIM's program sessions that have taken place over ASIM's growing-up years.

8

Miscellany

Avocations, Amusements, Anecdotes

A reliable sign of individual maturity, psychologists tell us, is the capacity to lead a balanced life, to pursue an appropriate mixture of work and fun. Any recounting of what ASIM leaders have accomplished stands the risk of making them sound like single-minded obsessives, dedicated only to working hard.

The truth is, of course, that ASIM shakers and movers differ little from other partakers of the human condition. Doubtless they work a little harder than most, and perhaps they have a somewhat more focused sense of purpose. But, being human, they have their share of idiosyncrasies. And they have found the saving grace of taking time to relax and have fun.

The Society's second president, Bert Persons, was unwilling to fly in airplanes; as a result, his stewardship had to be carried out from his office in Durham, and the not-too-affluent ASIM had to hire a part-time secretary to assist him. ASIM's late sixties' president, Robert Long, refused to compromise with his conviction that steak was the best—the only—entree; it could be "New York cut" but had better come from the Great Plains. Neither Malcolm Watts nor Clyde Greene would countenance imported wine; it is likely that they (along with other provincial patriots like Bullock, Molyneaux, Bristow and Wilbur) would have asked for a Napa Valley vintage even if the Board had met in Paris.

Although many ASIM officers and Trustees have devoted their leisure hours to conventional sports like golf, tennis and jogging, or to traditional hobbies like woodworking, painting and choral singing, a number have been less conventional. On the current Board, for instance, there is a writer of short stories (Bristow), a model train buff (Farrington), and an antique car owner (Abrums).

Personal habit patterns have been inconsistent. Years ago, Board meetings were often held in a cloud of blue tobacco smoke. As the

Surgeon General's admonition against cigarettes took hold, several patterns of response could be discerned among ASIM leaders: some capitulated, giving up tobacco completely; others were defiant, insisting on their right to continue to use coffin nails; in the middle were those who, wanting to have their tobacco and smoke it too, resorted to pipes, regular cigars, or (in the pretense of not really smoking) small cigars. The mix of persuasions varied from time to time, but, in 1970, the wily, and evangelically antitobacco Richard Wilbur found his chance and proffered a resolution that would forbid smoking of any kind during Board sessions; the resolution passed by a narrow margin and is still a rule of the Board—although it is honored, depending on the habits of the presiding officer, to the letter or in the breach.

Almost since the beginning, it has been customary for the ASIM president to occupy a suite in the meeting hotel, and it has been the custom for Board members to repair to the suite for a libation—often before lunch, always before dinner, and at times (unless the door is locked, either by a tired president or a solicitous president's wife) before bed. While the presidential suite is a site for relaxation, a refreshing drink, chitchat and the telling of stories, it is also a place for getting accomplished some of the real business of ASIM. Off in one corner, a subcommittee of three persons meets, working at its assignment to change from muddy to clear the language of a Board report to the House. In another spot, the President is buttonholing a prospect, "I'm asking you to chair this task force. . . ." Over here, a cluster of Trustees is arguing about the subtly different meanings of the words "posture," "position," and "policy." And over there, the President-Elect is waxing enthusiastic, "Wouldn't it be great if we could . . ." to which a past president wearily responds with a deflating "Well, we tried it and it didn't work because. . . ."

To be sure, decisive votes are taken only at formal Board sessions. But it is at the President's suite that concepts are developed, positions jelled, waverers won over, and opponents worn down—all this accomplished so that the voice at the formal sessions is nearly always unanimous. A cynic might say that thus is ASIM's consensus developed—snort and suite.

It should not be thought that formal meetings of the Board are always the rational, balanced, business-like sessions that Dorothy Titland's estimable minutes make them sound. The degree of orderliness depends mostly on the presiding officer and whether he is compulsive or laissez-faire about achieving the delicate balance between "letting all views be heard" and "getting on with the agenda." A desirable objective, of course, is to stymie the deplorable habit of Trustees discussing the important issues in haste and the trivial ones in depth, instead of vice versa. An obligatory strategy is to quell the loquacious and stimulate the laconic, to awaken the napper and quiet the overenthusiastic.

One way to grease the whole process is by calling on one or more responsible Board members to speed things along: during the late sixties the Trustee tandem of Painter and Wilbur could be counted on to expedite matters through rapid-fire and carefully-timed interjections—"So move," "Second," "Call the question."

Frank Riddick's quick brain found time at Board meetings both to keep track of what was going on and to produce some fertile inventions. His specialty was the composition of short-order limericks—always irreverent and frequently bawdy—on any subject or person, especially the pretentious or sanctimonious; the product, passed surreptitiously around the table to fellow Trustees, would inevitably break up the reader, not to mention the flow of business. Unfortunately, these works of art cannot today be found in ASIM's archives; one's memory suggests that most would not have been suitable for a family history anyhow.

It was Riddick and one or two other semantically oriented pundits on the Board who found themselves irked by the blandness of the standard parliamentary and management jargon that is universally affected by members of committees and boards. They proposed that more lively—and accurate—alternatives should be used; instead of "approved as amended," substitute "approved as obfuscated" or "approved as emasculated." The faint praise approbation that is so often awarded to a report ready for filing—"accepted with commendation" should be changed, these heretics suggested, to a more truthful phrase—"accepted with condemnation."

Painter's penchant for orderly structure resulted in the presentation to him by his fellow Trustees of a dubious commemorative award. It was his wont to display things—a planning report, a presidential address, a proposed Council/committee table or organization—in a carefully thought-out way, at the very least in a chart or table, but preferably in the form of overlapping Venn circles, or, even better, in simulated boxes or spheres. To point up this obsessional pattern to Painter, his fellow Trustees designed, constructed and presented to him an elaborate, Rube Goldberg, three-dimensional plastic model, full of evident cubes, spheres, pyramids, and other geometric shapes. The accompanying scroll—replete with references to ellipses, rhomboids, oblate spheroids and black holes—has also disappeared from ASIM archives—but perhaps can still be found, along with the red-ribboned contraption, occupying a place of honor (?) in the Painter trophy room.

It was this same Painter—apparently undaunted by the demonstration of the Board's feelings about his foible—who gave birth to the most visible and perpetual symbol of ASIM's lack of stodginess. Bothered by the tendency of Trustees to belabor inconsequentials and to skip over key issues, and searching for a device to keep them focused on the real business at hand, he chanced upon a joke going around at the time, the punch line of which was "When you're up to your ass in alligators, don't forget that your initial objective is to drain the swamp."

Immediately, the inventive Painter imagination went to work. In short order, he created an exclusive club—the Ancient Elliptical Order of Alligators (AEOA), designed a scroll as an award certificate, and arranged for a ceremonial occasion for the presentation of the honor to his fellow Trustees (all of whom, in his eyes, were fully deserving of the honor). At the ceremony, the awardees received not only the scroll (made of paper, alligator skin being so expensive), but also a small silver pin—yes, in the shape of an alligator—for proud display in the recipient's lapel.

Since its founding in 1970, the AEOA has become an institution. Sooner or later—usually sooner—all Trustees merit the honor; so do ASIM's top staffers, perhaps out of contagion. In 1980, in a grand gesture, all of ASIM's pre-1970 past presidents were given the award after retrospective review of their performance. And a small number of non-ASIMers—mostly a few AMA and Washington bigwigs—can wear the coveted silver alligator.

There has been talk of secret grips (but how do alligators shake hands?), of special libations (Gatorade and what?), and other expansions on the original theme. But most members of the Order are satisfied with the way things are now, with the simple annual award ceremony to add a few more deserving recipients to the ranks of those possessing the exclusive privilege of wearing that lapel pin.

What that silver alligator stands for, it turns out, is much more than an ongoing gag, an elite "in" joke. It signifies more than just a community of interests or a continuing camaraderie, although both of those exist. It symbolizes for its wearers, in the end, a memory of past travails, a joint sense of present purpose, and a common vision of the future—for themselves and their beloved ASIM.

9

The 25th Year

Audit of Actions

How does a mature organization—a thoroughly adult one like ASIM—comport itself? One way to answer that question is to take a snapshot, or perhaps a stop-shot movie, of its most recent year. It doesn't matter that the Society's 25th year, because of last year's Bylaws change in the date of the Annual Meeting, happens to be one-third longer than usual; it still manages to portray accurately the remarkable range and diversity of this energetic organization.

The "year" began in Washington in mid-May 1980, when 102 delegates and 30 alternates, representing 47 components and nine subspecialty societies, were seated to consider 25 Board reports, 34 resolutions, and a sprinkling of officer speeches, memorial resolutions, and special reports. Out of the deliberations taking place there (including one increasing annual dues from $100 to $125) would come a host of new policies and new programs.

The Board, charged with implementing House policy and with running the Society between House meetings, met in late August in New Mexico, in November in Florida, in March in New Orleans, and July in Wyoming; the Executive Committee had three additional meetings.

What kinds of activities were carried out during and between these meetings on behalf of ASIM and its members?

1. ASIM continued to pay attention to the national political and legislative scene:
   a. The Board took cognizance of the national election and of the pendulum swing in political philosophy accompanying it.
   b. The Board appointed task forces to review the Society's position on major health care issues—PSROs, HSAs, Medicare, "pro-competition" legislation.
   c. Thereafter, the Board reviewed, and in some cases revised, its positions and policies, concluding that the Society was prepared for the variety of eventualities which might arise.
   d. The Society's lobbyist made contact with important persons in the Executive Branch and on Capitol Hill.

   e. Selected officers met with top officials in the Health Care Financing Administration, to discuss Current Procedural Terminology, cognitive services, and other topics.
2. ASIM continued to pay attention to other major, ongoing health care issues:
   a. The Task Force on Cost Effectiveness continued its studies, developed a special project on purchasing drugs in hospitals, and agreed to serve as a major participant in an AMA conference on cost containment for specialty societies.
   b. A committee prepared, and the Board approved, a position statement on care for geriatric patients.
   c. Working through a task force, a major effort was initiated to point up the disparity between reimbursement for cognitive and for procedural services. A "white paper" was published and widely distributed as the opening round in a long-term campaign to correct that disparity.
   d. The Board decided to pursue negotiations with third-party payors, the object being to secure fairer reimbursement for internists' services.
   e. The Board endorsed a Federated Council for Internal Medicine-generated statement on "The Internist."
   f. A lengthy list of specific responses to each recommendation of the Graduate Medical Education National Advisory Committee (GMENAC) report was approved by the Board.
3. ASIM devoted time to improving its internal processes:
   a. The McManis Report (prepared by a professional management consultant) relating to staff functions was received and many of its recommendations were implemented.
   b. The Board authorized the purchase of a word processor and of a minicomputer for use in the headquarters office, in order to improve the communications function and the processing of membership and financial data.
   c. A lease was signed for a larger and better-situated headquarters office in downtown Washington, the move to take place later this year.
   d. Members of the Board discussed at length the Society's objectives, making revisions so as to make them more realistic, and reinforced the system of assigning Trustees to manage each of the objectives.
   e. The Board reviewed the workings of the important Function and Budget Committee, and further refined the role it plays in implementing the Society's short- and long-term plans.
   f. The Board clarified the function of the foundation—

ASIM/SEREF—approved projects proposed by it, and reviewed the role of its task force.

4. ASIM continued to pay attention to the needs of its members:
   a. The Board endorsed a multi-part Practice Information System, generated by the Ambulatory Care Committee with the help of MILCOM (a nationally prominent medical systems company), to be marketed to members for use in their practices.
   b. The Board approved a policy statement about patient access to medical records:
   c. A committee was charged with developing a series of malpractice education/prevention articles.
   d. The Board approved a committee-developed form for hospital patient referral/consult requests.
   e. A position on periodic health evaluations was reworded and sharpened.
   f. A committee was authorized to develop an educational program on computer applications in office practice.
   g. A "white paper" was developed on the new JCAH quality assurance standard.
   h. Guidelines were revised and issued on "Electrocardiogram Interpretation in the Hospital Setting."
   i. The Board took steps to clarify its position on medical specialty profiling, a problem troubling two component societies.
5. ASIM continued to relate to other medical and professional organizations:
   a. Liaison meetings were held with the American Academy of Family Physicians, the American College of Radiology, and the College of American Pathologists.
   b. The Private Initiative in Quality Assurance (PIQuA) project, cosponsored by ASIM, ACP, and the American Hospital Association, entered into a field test phase.
6. ASIM, as usual, spent time on its internal affairs:
   a. A membership campaign was initiated in various locales, including one in New York City called the Manhattan Project.
   b. The Investment Committee continued its laudatory handling of the various Society funds under its aegis.
   c. Two perennial issues—the possibility of creating a life membership category and the pros and cons of having House speaker/vice speaker positions—were aired, both receiving a negative reaction once again.
7. ASIM devoted time discussing a wide range of other topics, including:
   a. Financial support of medical education
   b. The possible future need for physician unions

c. Physician extenders
d. Wholistic medicine
e. State legislation of physician relicensure

Although impressive, the items displayed above by no means exhaust the list of activities which took place under the Society's banner during the year.

Item: Each of ASIM's 51 component societies had its own roster of activities, including meetings, newsletters, special projects, and liaison efforts.

Item: ASIM communicated with its more than 17,000 members through ten informative *Internist* issues and through 12 four-page *Intercoms,* and with component leaders through 12 *Component Society Officers Bulletins*.

Item: Each of ASIM's officers and Trustees pursued a hectic schedule of Board meetings, symposia, conferences, component gatherings, speech-making, etc.

Item: ASIM staff members prepared memoranda, attended conferences, travelled to component meetings, and performed dozens of other tasks designed to advance ASIM.

Probably no one person in ASIM today, not President Farrington, not Executive Vice President Ramsey, can know *all* that goes on under the aegis of ASIM and its components. The threads are too diverse and their interweaving too complex for anyone to get more than a general idea of the entire tapestry of ASIM activities.

Nor can any one individual (an officer, a top staffer) or any one group (the Board, the House, the staff) be said to be primarily responsible for making the organization work.

The fact is that ASIM works because of the aggregate input of hundreds of individuals and dozens of groups, each supplying, to a greater or lesser degree, a fragment of the total remarkable effort that is ASIM.

POSTLUDE

ASIM's Future

Ad Astra

ASIM'S Future
Ad Astra

Futurists—persons who predict what will happen down the road—are much in vogue these days. Such people, whether they are individual crystal ball gazers or teams of computer-assisted think tank experts, can be hired to project current trends and to make calculated guesses about the future of almost anything. Without question, prophets could be found willing, for money, to take a stab at what will happen to ASIM in its next 25 years.

But the suspicion arises that predicting the future is a dubious pastime, particularly in the volatile health care field. One thing that has become evident during recent decades is that actions taken now (however well-meaning) will produce unanticipated results down the road, ripple effects that, whether they turn out to be salutary or disastrous, were simply not foreseen.

If prophesy is so dubious and the future so murky, is it therefore impossible to say anything meaningful about ASIM's future? The thought here is that the Society has a number of things going for it, some attributes that tend to give it staying power.

For one thing, there is the homogeneity of ASIM's membership. Serving—as it nearly exclusively does—the needs of practicing internists, ASIM has a sharp, definable mission and an identifiable commonality of interest. As long as young internists continue to go out into the world of practice, they will continue to look for an organization to represent them, both for their local, practice-related problems and to uphold their interests at the national policy-making level.

Another plus lies in ASIM's grassroots decision-making process. The checks and balances inherent in a House of Delegates/Board of Trustees structure breeds a certain stability and tends to increase the likelihood that organizational positions will be rational ones and that decisions will be taken with deliberate balance. The net effect is credibility, in the eyes of members and of the outside world.

Another, and closely related, attribute is what might be called the ASIM method—the transfer of the energetic, problem-solving approach used by internists in their care of patients to the resolution of difficult problems in the social, economic and political arenas of health care.

Finally, ASIM has momentum going for it. The simple truth is that the Society, over the course of 25 years, has come to grips with nearly all the important health care issues, that it has a policy or position on most of them, and that, for many of them, it has ongoing programmatic activities. In addition, ASIM "graduates," inculcated with its ap-

proach, today hold important positions throughout the health care field.

Another test of an organization's ability to endure is to ask the question: "If it were not on the scene today, would someone have to invent it?" In certain quarters, the question would probably receive a negative answer. The AMA is championing its own preeminent role in medical affairs, and while it has always enjoyed friendly relationships with ASIM, would not be likely to go out of its way to create such a strong specialty organization. Similarly, the American College of Physicians, lately committed to involvement in the social, economic, and political aspects of health, would be unlikely to welcome a rival internal medicine organization into the arena, the arguments being that the internist's method can be delivered as well by College internists, and that grassroots process and federation structure are either unimportant or could come along later.

The view here is that a health care world without ASIM in it would be sadly diminished, in many small aspects and a few big ones. The guess is that, if no ASIM existed, there would be tomorrow, as there were 25 years ago, groups of internists meeting together to discuss mutual problems and deciding that a national organization is needed to work effectively on behalf of internists and their patients.

It's more of a guess than a prediction: ASIM will continue to pursue its vigorous path; it will not merely survive, it will flourish.

APPENDIX

Historical Listings

Appropriate Appreciation

1

ASIM Presidents

Lewis T. Bullock, MD, Los Angeles, California	1957–58
* Elbert L. Persons, MD, Durham, North Carolina	1958–59
Clark C. Goss, MD, Laguna Hills, California	1959–60
Stewart P. Seigle, MD, Hartford, Connecticut	1960–61
* Ross V. Taylor, MD, Jackson, Michigan	1961–62
Charles K. Donegan, MD, St. Petersburg, Florida	1962–63
Maxwell G. Berry, MD, Kansas City, Missouri	1963–64
Malcolm S.M. Watts, MD, San Francisco, California	1964–65
Robert E. Westlake, MD, Syracuse, New York	1965–66
Wendell B. Gordon, MD, Pittsburgh, Pennsylvania	1966–67
James J. Feffer, MD, Washington, D.C.	1967–68
Robert S. Long, MD, Omaha, Nebraska	1968–69
Clyde C. Greene, Jr., MD, San Francisco, California	1969–70
Joseph T. Painter, MD, Houston, Texas	1970–71
Otto C. Page, MD, Portland, Oregon	1971–72
Edwin C. Evans, MD, Atlanta, Georgia	1972–73
William Campbell Felch, MD, Rye, New York	1973–74
Glenn Molyneaux, MD, San Francisco, California	1974–75
Ralph F. Reinfrank, MD, Hartford, Connecticut	1975–76
William R. Felts, MD, Washington, D.C.	1976–77
William P. Daines, MD, Ogden, Utah	1977–78
Ben D. Hall, MD, Johnson City, Tennessee	1978–79
James A. Collins, Jr., MD, Danville, Pennsylvania	1979–80
John F. Farrington, MD, Boulder, Colorado	1980–81

* Deceased

2

ASIM Trustees

Lewis T. Bullock, MD, Los Angeles, California	1957–1959
* Elbert L. Persons, MD, Durham, North Carolina	1957–1960
* Claude P. Callaway, MD, San Francisco, California	1957–1958
* Wallace M. Yater, MD, Washington, D.C.	1957–1960
Clark C. Goss, MD, Laguna Hills, California	1957–1961
Stewart P. Seigle, MD, Hartford, Connecticut	1957–1962
George K. Wever, MD, Stockton, California	1957–1961
H. Marvin Pollard, MD, Ann Arbor, Michigan	1958–1959
Clyde C. Greene, Jr., MD, San Francisco, California	1958–1971
Charles K. Donegan, MD, St. Petersburg, Florida	1959–1964
* L. Philip Longley, MD, Shaker Heights, Ohio	1959–1964
Henry J. Lehnhoff, MD, Omaha, Nebraska	1959–1962
* Ross V. Taylor, MD, Jackson, Michigan	1960–1963
Robert E. Westlake, MD, Syracuse, New York	1960–1967
* Howard F. Root, MD, Boston, Massachusetts	1960–1963
Malcolm S.M. Watts, MD, San Francisco, California	1961–1966
Maxwell G. Berry, MD, Kansas City, Missouri	1961–1965
Wendell B. Gordon, MD, Delray Beach, Florida	1961–1968
Robert L. Gilbert, MD, La Crosse, Wisconsin	1962–1968
James J. Feffer, MD, Washington, D.C.	1962–1969
Robert S. Long, MD, Omaha, Nebraska	1962–1970
Frank P. Foster, MD, Hanover, New Hampshire	1963–1968
Otto C. Page, MD, Portland, Oregon	1963–1973
* Bert M. Bullington, MD, Saginaw, Michigan	1963–1964
Carter Smith, MD, Atlanta, Georgia	1964–1967
Peter J. Talso, MD, Hines, Illinois	1964–1967
Charles Weller, MD, Larchmont, New York	1964–1968
Joseph T. Painter, MD, Houston, Texas	1965–1972
Richard S. Wilbur, MD, Chicago, Illinois	1966–1970
Edwin C. Evans, MD, Atlanta, Georgia	1967–1972
Blaine Z. Hibbard, MD, Kansas City, Missouri	1967–1973
Charley J. Smyth, MD, Denver, Colorado	1967–1970
Charles F. Downing, MD, Decatur, Illinois	1968–1972
William Campbell Felch, MD, Rye, New York	1968–1975
Horace H. Hodges, MD, Charlotte, North Carolina	1968–1971
Ralph F. Reinfrank, MD, Hartford, Connecticut	1968–1977
Glenn Molyneaux, MD, San Francisco, California	1969–1976

William R. Felts, MD, Washington, D.C.	1969–1978
Frank A. Riddick, Jr., MD, New Orleans, Louisiana	1970–1976
William P. Daines, MD, Ogden, Utah	1970–1979
Ben D. Hall, MD, Johnson City, Tennessee	1971–1980
William A. Millhon, MD, Columbus, Ohio	1971–1979
James A. Collins, Jr., MD, Danville, Pennsylvania	1972–1981
Mervin Shalowitz, MD, Skokie, Illinois	1972–1980
John F. Farrington, MD, Boulder, Colorado	1973–
Carmault B. Jackson, Jr., MD, San Antonio, Texas	1973–1976
John V. Verner, Jr., MD, Lakeland, Florida	1974–1976
Monte Malach, MD, Brooklyn, New York	1975–
John D. Abrums, MD, Albuquerque, New Mexico	1976–
Lonnie R. Bristow, MD, San Pablo, California	1976–
T. Reginald Harris, MD, Shelby, North Carolina	1976–
Michael P. Mehr, MD, Marshfield, Wisconsin	1976–1978
C. Burns Roehrig, MD, Boston, Massachusetts	1977–
N. Thomas Connally, MD, Washington, D.C.	1978–
F. Warren Tingley, MD, Arlington, Texas	1978–
Robert L. Hare, MD, Portland, Oregon	1979–
Paul S. Metzger, MD, Columbus, Ohio	1979–
Emanuel Abraham, MD, Neptune, New Jersey	1980–
Joseph A. Sentkeresty, MD, Grand Rapids, Michigan	1980–

* Deceased

3

Distinguished Internists of the Year

Dwight L. Wilbur, MD, San Francisco, California	1969
* Wallace Mason Yater, MD, Washington, D.C.	1970
Roberta F. Fenlon, MD, San Francisco, California	1971
Frank P. Foster, MD, West Lebanon, New Hampshire	1972
John Ruskin Graham, MD, Aurora, Colorado	1973
Jere W. Annis, MD, Lakeland, Florida	1974
E. Harvey Estes, MD, Durham, North Carolina	1975
Saul J. Farber, MD, New York, New York	1976
Edward C. Rosenow, Jr., MD, Philadelphia, Pennsylvania	1977
Katherine H. Borkovich, MD, Baltimore, Maryland	1978
Charley J. Smyth, MD, Denver, Colorado	1979
Lowell H. Steen, MD, Hammond, Indiana	1980
Frank A. Riddick, Jr., MD, New Orleans, Louisiana	1981

* Deceased

4

Young Internists of the Year

Frank A. Riddick, Jr., MD, New Orleans, Louisiana	1969
Alfred D. Biggs, Jr., MD, Kansas City, Missouri	1970
Joseph G. Katterhagen, MD, Tacoma, Washington	1971
James L. Borland, MD, Jacksonville, Florida	1972
Lawrence M. Cutchin, MD, Tarboro, North Carolina	1973
Robert K. Maddock, Jr., MD, Salt Lake City, Utah	1974
N. Thomas Connally, MD, Washington, D.C.	1976
James G. Nuckolls, MD, Galax, Virginia	1977
Peter G. Tuteur, MD, St. Louis, Missouri	1980
Michael C. Perry, MD, Columbia, Missouri	1981

5

Component Societies of the Year

Florida Society of Internal Medicine	1969
Massachusetts Society of Internal Medicine	1970
Pennsylvania Society of Internal Medicine	1971
Colorado Society of Internal Medicine	1972
New York State Society of Internal Medicine	1973
North Carolina Society of Internal Medicine	1974
Utah Society of Internal Medicine	1975
Oregon Society of Internal Medicine	1976
New Jersey Society of Internal Medicine	1977
South Carolina Society of Internal Medicine	1978
Georgia Society of Internal Medicine	1979
Wisconsin Society of Internal Medicine	1980
Virginia Society of Internal Medicine	1981

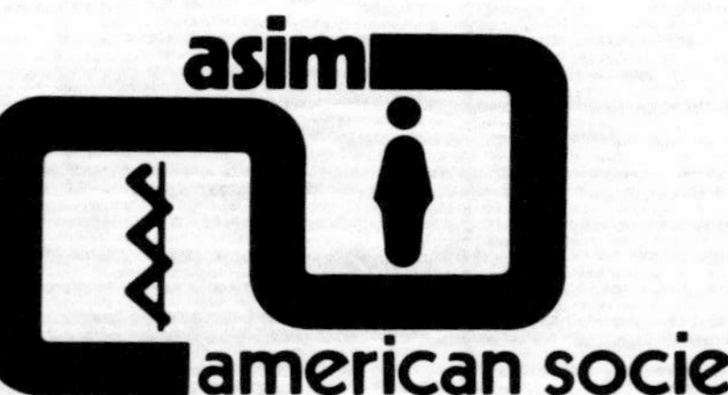

american society of internal medicine

October 1980

Dear Members and Friends of ASIM,

It is our pleasure to provide you with a copy of Aspiration & Achievement, the story of the American Society of Internal Medicine from 1956-81, by ASIM past presidents William Campbell Felch, MD, and Clyde C. Greene, Jr., MD.

This informal history chronicles the birth and growth of ASIM as the practicing internist's advocate in the socioeconomic and political aspects of medical practice.

We invite your reflections, recollections and responses

Sincerely,

John F. Farrington, MD
President, 1980-81

Lonnie R. Bristow, MD
President, 1981-82

2550 M STREET NW · SUITE 620 · WASHINGTON, DC 20037 · TELEPHONE (202) 659-0330